Non-invasive Surrogate Markers of Atherosclerosis

Non-invasive Surrogate Markers of Atherosclerosis

Edited by

Steven B Feinstein MD

Echocardiography Laboratory
Section of Cardiology
Rush University Medical Center
Chicago, IL
USA

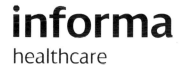

©2008 Informa UK Ltd

First published in the United Kingdom in 2008 by Informa Healthcare, Telephone House, 69–77 Paul Street, London EC2A 4LQ. Informa Healthcare is a trading division of Informa UK Ltd. Registered Office: 37/41 Mortimer Street, London W1T 3JH. Registered in England and Wales number 1072954.

Tel: +44 (0)20 7017 5000
Fax: +44 (0)20 7017 6699
Website: www.informahealthcare.com

A CIP record for this book is available from the British Library.
Library of Congress Cataloging-in-Publication Data

Data available on application

ISBN-10: 1 84184 635 X
ISBN-13: 978 1 84184 635 4

Distributed in North and South America by
Taylor & Francis
6000 Broken Sound Parkway, NW, (Suite 300)
Boca Raton, FL 33487, USA

Within Continental USA
Tel: 1 (800) 272 7737; Fax: 1 (800) 374 3401
Outside Continental USA
Tel: (561) 994 0555; Fax: (561) 361 6018
Email: orders@crcpress.com

Book orders in the rest of the world

Paul Abrahams
Tel: +44 207 017 4036
Email: bookorders@informa.com

Composition by Cepha Imaging Pvt Ltd, Bangalore, India.
Printed and bound in India by Replika Press, PVT Ltd.

Contents

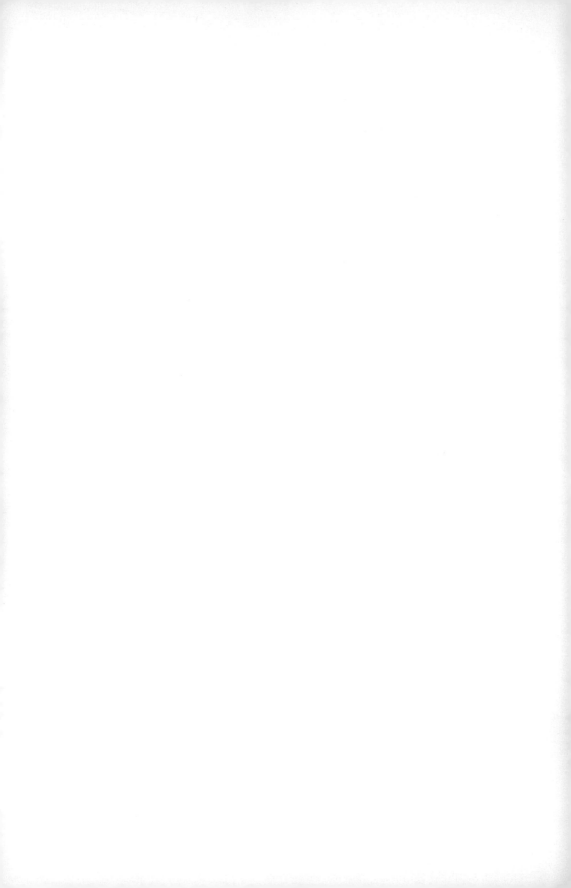

Contributors

STEPHAN ACHENBACH MD
Department of Cardiology
University of Erlangen
Erlangen
Germany

BARBARA C BIEDERMANN MD
University Department of Medicine
Kantonsspital Bruderholz
Bruderholz
Switzerland

FOLKERT J TEN CATE MD PHD
Department of Cardiology
Thoraxcenter
Erasmus MC
Rotterdam
The Netherlands

MICHAEL H DAVIDSON MD
Section of Cardiology
University of Chicago
Chicago, IL
USA

STEVEN B FEINSTEIN MD
Echocardiography Laboratory
Section of Cardiology
Rush University Medical Center
Chicago, IL
USA

MARCEL L GELEIJNSE MD PHD
Department of Cardiology
Thoraxcenter
Erasmus MC
Rotterdam
The Netherlands

BOUDEWIJN J KRENNING MD
Department of Cardiology
Thoraxcenter
Erasmus MC
Rotterdam
The Netherlands

PHILIP R LIEBSON MD
Cardiology and Preventive Medicine
Rush University Medical College
Chicago, IL
USA

ATTILA NEMES MD PHD
2ⁿᵈ Department of Medicine
Cardiology Center
University of Szeged
Szeged
Hungary

FRANCESCO PIZZUTO MD
Department of Cardiology
University of Rome 'Tor Vergata'
Rome
Italy

OSAMA II SOLIMAN MD
Department of Cardiology
Thoraxcenter
Erasmus MC
Rotterdam
The Netherlands

WILLEM B VLETTER MSC
Department of Cardiology
Thoraxcenter
Erasmus MC
Rotterdam
The Netherlands

PAOLO VOCI MD PHD
Department of Cardiology
University of Rome 'Tor Vergata'
Rome
Italy

Preface

An aging, overweight, sedentary baby boomer population is under siege. Approximately 58 million people die from cardiovascular diseases each year, nearly 1.2 million from heart attacks and 700,000 from strokes in the United States alone. Moreover, against a backdrop of world-wide pan-epidemics of obesity and metabolic syndrome, nearly one-third of the American population is at risk for developing diabetes, which is linked to cardiovascular disease and increased risk of premature death. The baby boomers' children also are at risk of developing premature cardiovascular disease, which is due in part to their inactive lifestyles and social behaviors. These uncomfortable statistics are likely to worsen in the future.

Therefore, it is critical to accelerate the wide-spread implementation of non-invasive imaging technology that reliably identifies surrogate markers of atherosclerosis and permits the detection of at-risk populations. This technology provides guideposts for instituting therapy and monitoring clinical responses.

Our book, *Non-Invasive Surrogate Markers of Atherosclerosis*, provides a survey of wide-ranging technology that can help physicians identify at-risk patients. My colleagues have synthesized their latest work in this field, and present it in an exciting and useful format. I am indebted to all of the contributors to this book for their tireless devotion to the advancement of medical care. On behalf of all of us, I also want to express sincere appreciation to our families and friends for their support, encouragement and belief in our work.

We all hope that this book will provide useful guidance that ultimately will help patients lead longer, healthier lives.

Steven Feinstein MD
Chicago, February 2008

1

Echocardiography: left ventricular hypertrophy and atherosclerosis

Philip R Liebson

INTRODUCTION

The focus of this chapter is an analysis of the interaction of coronary and peripheral atherosclerosis and left ventricular (LV) structure, specifically, LV hypertrophy (LVH). This includes factors related to coronary blood flow (CBF) and the consequences of LVH in patients with coronary artery disease. We will not cover the consequences of inadequate coronary flow per se, such as LV wall motion abnormalities, or morphologic changes such as ventricular aneurysm formation secondary to myocardial infarction.

LV MASS AND ATHEROSCLEROTIC DISEASE

The structure and function of the LV wall reflect the resultant of the stresses exerted on the myocardium, the constitution of myocardial tissue itself (muscle/fibrous tissue ratio), and the coronary vasculature supplying the muscle (Table 1.1). Atherosclerosis of the coronary vasculature can induce LV regional wall motion abnormalities. Atherosclerosis of the aorta induces decreased arterial elastance and can affect the systolic stress on the LV wall, leading to LVH. This may be seen in elderly subjects with isolated systolic hypertension. Although coronary artery disease (CAD) can lead to compensatory LVH in non-involved myocardium when ischemic segments are hypokinetic or dyskinetic, pathophysiologic LVH is most commonly associated with hypertension and the volume overload seen in obesity, aside from valvular abnormalities. Both coronary atherosclerosis and the process of pathologic LVH per se can be associated with interstitial fibrosis leading to diastolic stiffness. In large population studies, LV mass is independently determined by systolic blood pressure, stroke volume, contractility, body mass index, and aortic root diameter. Finally, LVH can affect

Table 1.1   The association of LV mass and atherosclerotic disease

Factors related to atherosclerosis increasing LV mass

Hypertension
Stiff aorta- increased augmentation index
Increased angiotensin II
Obesity
Insulin

Correlations of increased LV mass with atherosclerosis

Coronary artery calcium
Carotid intimal-medial thickness
Aortic atherosclerosis
Atherosclerotic renal vascular disease (microalbuminuria)
Peripheral vascular disease

Effects of increased LV mass on coronary blood flow

Increased coronary flow reserve
• cardiomyocytes
• fibrosis

coronary flow reserve (CFR), increasing the adverse effects of coronary artery atherosclerosis.

Myocardial regional wall stress/CBF differences are present through the thickness of the myocardial wall. The endocardium is more vulnerable than the epicardium to myocardial ischemia, since systolic tension and resulting CBF are higher. Because of the orientation of the circumferential and meridional musculature, the inner half of the myocardial wall characteristically thickens more than the outer half.[1] This increases the vulnerability of the inner half of the myocardial wall to systolic dysfunction resulting from myocardial ischemia.

Efforts have been made to assess CBF or coronary atherosclerosis by echocardiography (echo). Studies have focused on the left anterior descending (LAD) and posterior descending (PD) coronary arteries.[2] Visualization of the coronary vessels is accomplished by using a high resolution transducer with the transducer placed above the cardiac apex and focused on the proximal field. The mid-distal LAD or PD is visualized by color Doppler and pulsed Doppler velocities are determined. Adenosine is particularly useful to measure coronary flow velocity reserve since it is a pure microvascular dilator and does not alter the caliber of the epicardial coronary artery.[2]

SIGNIFICANCE OF LVH

Numerous studies have assessed the prevalence and adverse prognosis of LVH.[3-7] In a general population, LVH increases with age and may be present in as many as 19% of a general population aged 17–90, using echo criteria.[3] In hypertensive patients, its prevalence may vary from 20 to 50%.[8,9] Increases in quartiles of LV mass even below levels of LVH are associated with increased risk for CV disease events, estimated in one epidemiologic study as an approximately 50% increase in risk for each 50 g/m increase in LV mass/height index in men or women.[4]

Using the NHANES II Mortality Study results (1976–1992), Brown et al reported that persons with LVH were twice as likely to die of CAD after adjustment for hypertension and covariates.[5] Moreover, the absence of hypertension did not affect mortality differences in those with LVH vs non-LVH. In a study of 2461 patients initially diagnosed with CAD by angiography, patients with LVH had a 56% greater 3-year mortality than those without LVH after adjusting for other clinical risk factors.[6] The diagnostic criteria for LVH, either by echo or ECG, predict mortality independently of each other.[7] In another angiographic study for assessment of CAD, geometric remodeling patterns of LVH differentially affected mortality risk, with concentric hypertrophy (increased wall thickness/LV chamber radius) associated with a higher risk than eccentric hypertrophy (normal thickness/radius ratio) and normal geometry.[10] In patients with CAD, concentric hypertrophy was associated with a relative risk of 2.2 for cardiac death compared with normal geometry. A previous analysis of hypertensive patients without CAD showed a similar increased risk for cardiac mortality with concentric hypertrophy.[11]

The anatomic association of LV mass with coronary atherosclerosis has been determined using electron beam tomographic (EBT) scanning in conjunction with echo assessment. Correlations for coronary artery calcium with LV mass have been found in young adults,[12] and in a group of hypertensive patients.[13]

The pathogenesis of LVH, although influenced by LV wall stress, is associated with processes that are also increased in the coronary vasculature to propagate atherosclerosis. For example, angiotensin II plays an important role in the induction of LVH[14] as well as in atherogenesis. Inflammatory markers, such as vascular adhesion molecule-1 (sVCAM-1), are increased in LVH as in atherosclerosis.[15] The fibrosis seen in LVH may be due to normal or abnormal collagen production. It is possible that reactive fibrosis is triggered in part by myocardial ischemia.[14]

LV mass increases have been found to influence endothelium-dependent vasodilation of forearm blood flow, independent of blood pressure increases.[16] LVH may also be associated with endothelial dysfunction in the coronary vessels.[17,18]

Ultrasound has been used to evaluate cardiac fibrosis in hypertensives using the technique of real-time integrated backscatter analysis, which provides information on cyclic variation of backscatter during the cardiac cycle. In LVH, especially in hypertension, increased accumulation of fibrillar collagens I and III develops, increasing myocardial stiffness and influencing CFR by perivascular infiltration.[19] Increased serum levels of carboxy-terminal propeptide of procollagen type I (PIP) appear to correlate with myocardial fibrosis, and also with decreased cyclic variation of integrated backscatter, suggesting an approach by echo for assessment of cardiac fibrotic changes associated with LVH.

METABOLIC CONSIDERATIONS

As indicated above, metabolic factors associated with the development and persistence of LVH may also be common in atherogenesis. Some of these findings in LVH are associated primarily with hypertension, of which LVH is highly correlated. For example, a cross-sectional study of patients attending a hypertension clinic compared with healthy normotensive controls showed an increase in inflammatory and thrombogenic factors such as P-selectin, plasmin activator-inhibitor-1 (PAI-1), von Willebrand factor, Lp(a), and fibrinogen, all of which are metabolically active in atherosclerosis, involving platelet activation, endothelial dysfunction, impaired fibrinolysis, and thrombogenesis.[20]

The myocardial G-protein receptors, including angiotensin and endothelin-1, regulate hypertrophic growth but are also active in processes leading to endothelial dysfunction and the production of reactive oxygen species (ROS).[21,22] Impaired endothelial regulation of relaxation seen in LVH appears to be associated with increased production of ROS, in part at least from increased NADP oxidase activity, expressed in both endothelial cells and myocytes.[23]

In hypertrophied myocytes, fatty acid oxidation is suppressed and glucose utilization increased, decreasing myocardial oxygen consumption/ATP generated.[24] It is interesting that a decrease in peroxisome proliferator-activator receptor gene α (PPARα) expression may be linked to the magnitude of LVH (CC genotype).[25] Moreover, hypertrophic stimuli may decrease PPARα in the cardiac myocytes within hours.[26,27] PPARγ- deficient mice have also been demonstrated to display exaggerated hypertrophic response to pressure overload.[28,29] There appears to be a parallel protective effect of PPARγ activity on modulation of hypertrophy and on limiting factors that could lead to increased atherogenesis such as increased insulin resistance, PAI-1 levels, C-reactive protein levels, and other inflammatory mediators.[30]

The effects of insulin on stimulating LVH may influence the high prevalence of LVH in type 2 diabetes. For example, Dawson et al demonstrated a prevalence of LVH in 71% of 500 type 2 diabetic patients although only 4% had systolic function abnormalities.[31] Insulin shows ex vivo evidence of growth effects on cardiomyocytes,[32] and levels are increased in type 2 diabetes. Insulin-like growth factor-II has also been shown to stimulate cardiac hypertrophy.[33] Another emerging mechanism is the link between obesity, diabetes, and LVH in relation to leptin activity.[34] Leptin is secreted by fat cells and acts on receptors in the hypothalamus to decrease food intake and increase expenditure. Leptin regulates the efficiency of insulin-mediated glucose metabolism. Levels are increased in obesity and hypertension. Leptin deficiency is associated with LVH in animal model studies.[35] Paradoxically, leptin levels can be increased in hypertension and obesity because of decreased leptin signaling, indicating a decreased receptor sensitivity. Associated insulin sensitivity decreases produced by increased food intake and obesity result in LVH and autonomic overactivity.[34] If leptin is administered in primary leptin deficiency, however, LVH is rapidly reduced.[35] Thus, insulin resistance, overweight, and hypertension, constituting elements of the metabolic syndrome and associated with increased risk for atherogenesis, are also associated with LVH.

The association of angiotensin II with atherogenesis and LVH through the AT_1 receptor must also be considered. Signaling through the AT_{1a} receptor activates multiple pathways which increase intracellular calcium, and mitogen-activated protein (MAP) among other substances, which lead to myocyte hypertrophy and inflammatory processes stimulating atherogenesis.[36]

LVH AND CORONARY HEMODYNAMICS

The impact of LVH on CBF is especially important with underlying coronary atherosclerosis since increased LV mass can affect CFR, which may also be compromised by a number of factors including epicardial coronary artery stenosis, wall thickening of the resistance arterioles, cardiomyocyte hypertrophy, perivascular and interstitial fibrosis, and reduced density of the arterioles.[37]

Some experimental and clinical studies have associated LVH with decreased CFR,[38,39] although the independent effect of LVH on CFR has been disputed by others.[40,41]

In support of the relation of LV mass to reduced CFR, Kozàkovà et al compared 64 untreated middle-aged hypertensive patients without significant coronary stenosis with normotensive volunteers.[38] Minimum coronary resistance was increased in hypertensive patients without LVH, but more so in those with LVH compared with normotensive individuals. In addition to lower coronary vasodilator capacity, LVH was associated with depressed LV wall mechanics and abnormal diastolic filling pattern. There is evidence that increased LV mass is related to increased arterial wall thickness,[42] possibly related to effects of angiotensin II.

On the other hand, in a study of 21 subjects with never treated hypertension without inducible myocardial ischemia, CFR was not significantly related to LV mass although reduced flow mediated coronary dilatation, an indication of endothelial dysfunction, varied inversely with LV mass.[40] Gimelli et al evaluated 50 untreated hypertensive patients and found that, although at baseline CBF was similar to that of normotensive subjects, CFR was decreased but did not correlate with LV mass.[41] However, there appeared to be areas of focal regional flow abnormalities in a group with a heterogeneous flow pattern, more common with increased LV mass. The conclusion from this study was that in hypertensive patients in general, there is a decrease in CFR that is not specifically determined by LV mass. However, regression of LVH has been shown to improve CFR.[43]

A study of 25 patients with hypertensive LVH and normal or mildly diseased coronary arteries with evidence for myocardial ischemia indicated that myocardial ischemia was dependent on the degree of intimal thickness, with or without plaque accumulation, and maximal vasodilating capacity of the resistance coronary arteries in relation to minimal coronary resistance.[44]

Besides the myocardial wall stress/CBF ratio, the efficiency of LV contraction may be affected by increased LV mass. A study of hypertensive men with or without LVH demonstrated that myocardial oxygen consumption per unit weight of myocardium is increased in those without LVH, as would be suggested by the increased wall stress, but is normal in those with LVH, which reflects the compensatory effects of LVH on maintaining normal wall stress.[45] However, the efficiency of the unit weight of myocardium is reduced, based upon the ratio of mean arterial pressure and cardiac output/myocardial oxygen consumption. It is presumed that the decrease in efficiency could predispose to heart failure. The significance of this finding with respect to CFR requires further examination.

There is evidence that LVH may influence coronary plaque disruption. One study implicated LV muscle mass > 270 g and heart rate > 80 beats/minute as independently correlated with plaque disruption.[46]

ARTERIAL STRUCTURE AND LVH

The presence of aortic atherosclerosis influences the systolic pressure and hence the development of LVH. On the other hand, the presence of LVH may be associated with changes in the arterial tree. For example, Roman et al evaluated arterial structure and function by carotid ultrasound and applanation tonometry in 271 unmedicated hypertensive patients and demonstrated increased arterial wall thickness in patients with concentric LVH compared with other LV remodeling patterns.[42]

It is to be expected that changes in the blood pressure may affect the LV as well as the peripheral arterial tree. An important consideration is the peripheral arterial effects on the augmentation index, which measures the contribution of the reflected pulse wave from the periphery through the arterial wall in late systole.[47] The wave is more rapidly transmitted in stiffer arteries; its importance is that the brachial arterial systolic pressure may be lower than the central aortic systolic pressure as a result of the augmentation wave.

Arterial stiffness has been documented to be associated with inflammatory diseases and with increasing circulating levels of C-reactive protein and IL-6 in a cross-sectional study.[48] It is possible that these biomarkers could implicate a corresponding risk for atherosclerosis and LVH, the latter as a consequence of increasing aortic stiffness. In hemodialysis patients with accelerated atherosclerosis and vascular calcification, LVH was detected in 75% of plaque positive patients.[49] In a large population of 1315 Chinese subjects, who were normotensive or had untreated hypertension, although systolic blood pressure contributed most to independent prediction of LV mass, inertia of blood in the ascending aorta on ejection was also an independent risk predictor.[50]

In an analysis of stiffening arterial effects on LV mass, it is difficult to separate blood pressure itself from the augmentation of end systolic stress due to returning pulse waves in the aortic wall in stiff arteries. Thus, pulse pressure becomes important in elderly adults, reflecting changes in the aortic wall, whereas hypertension in younger individuals reflects primarily changes in the peripheral microvasculature.[51]

SUMMARY

LVH is a strong risk factor for cardiovascular events. Although ECG can be useful for screening, it is less sensitive than echo evaluation, which is considered the gold standard for diagnosis, although requiring meticulous performance and measurement for accuracy. LVH is associated with decreased CFR, which adds to the coronary flow impairment in coronary atherosclerosis. In addition, LVH correlates with more peripheral manifestations of atherosclerosis such as increased carotid intimal-medial thickness and plaque, microalbuminuria, and aortic atherosclerosis. Its association with hypertension influences its prevalence in CHD, aortic, and peripheral vascular disease. Aortic atherosclerosis, in turn, may influence the development of LVH by increasing impedance to LV flow in systole. Evaluation of atherosclerosis should also include assessment for the presence of LVH.

REFERENCES

1. Shimizu G, Hirota Y, Kita Y et al. Left ventricular midwall mechanics in systemic arterial hypertension. Circulation 1991; 83: 1676–84.
2. Voci P, Pizzuto F, Romeo F. Coronary flow: a new asset for the echo lab? Eur Heart J 2004; 35: 1867–79.
3. Levy D, Anderson KM, Savage DD et al. Echocardiographically detected left ventricular hypertrophy: prevalence and risk factors. The Framingham Heart Study. Ann Int Med 1988; 108: 7.
4. Levy D, Garrison RJ, Savage DD et al. Prognostic implications of echocardiographically determined left ventricular mass in the Framingham Heart Study. N Engl J Med 1990; 322: 1561.
5. Brown DW, Giles WH, Croft JB. Left ventricular hypertrophy as a predictor of coronary heart disease mortality and the effect of hypertension. Am Heart J 2000; 140: 848–56.
6. East MA, Jollis JG, Nelson CL et al. The influence of left ventricular hypertrophy on survival in patients with coronary artery disease: do race and gender matter? J Am Coll Cardiol 2003; 41: 949–54.
7. Sundström J, Lind L, Ärnlöv J et al. Echocardiographic and electrocardiographic diagnoses of left ventricular hypertrophy predict mortality independently of each other in a population of elderly men. Circulation 2001; 103: 2346.
8. Hammond IW, Devereux RB, Alderman MH et al. The prevalence and correlates of echocardiographic left ventricular hypertrophy among employed patients with uncomplicated hypertension. J Am Coll Cardiol 1986; 7: 639–50.
9. Sukhija R, Aranow WS, Kakar P et al. Prevalence of echocardiographic left ventricular hypertrophy in persons with systemic hypertension, coronary artery disease, and peripheral arterial disease and in persons with systemic hypertension, coronary artery disease, and no peripheral arterial disease. Am J Cardiol 2005; 96: 825–26.
10. Ghali JK, Liao Y, Cooper RS. Influence of left ventricular geometric patterns on prognosis in patients with or without coronary artery disease. J Am Coll Cardiol 1998; 31: 1635.
11. Koren MJ, Devereux RB, Casale PN et al. Relation of left ventricular mass and geometry to morbidity and mortality in uncomplicated essential hypertension. Ann Int Med 1991; 114: 345.
12. Gardin JM, Iribarren C, Detrano RC et al. The relation of echocardiographic left ventricular mass, geometry and wall stress, and left atrial dimension to coronary calcium in young adults (The CARDIA study). Am J Cardiol 2005; 95: 626–9.
13. Altunkan S, Erdogan N, Altin L, Budoff MJ. Relation of coronary artery calcium to left ventricular mass and geometry in patients with essential hypertension. Blood Pressure Monitoring 2003; 8: 9–15.
14. Lorell BH, Carabello BA. Left ventricular hypertrophy. Pathogenesis, detection, and prognosis. Circulation 2000; 102: 470–9.
15. Kuroda YT, Komamura K, Tatsumi R et al. Vascular cell adhesion molecule-1 as a biochemical marker of left ventricular mass in patients with hypertension. Am J Hypertens 2001; 14: 868–72.
16. Perticone F, Ceravolo R, Pujia A et al. Prognostic significance of endothelial dysfunction in hypertensive patients. Circulation 2001; 104: 191.
17. Treasure CB, Klein L, Vita JA et al. Hypertension and left ventricular hypertrophy are associated with impaired endothelium-mediated relaxation in human coronary resistance vessels. Circulation 1993; 87: 86–93.
18. Houghton JL, Strogatz DS, Torosoff, MT et al. African-Americans with LVH demonstrate depressed sensitivity of the coronary microvasculature to structural relaxation. Hypertension 2003; 42: 269–76.
19. Schwartzkopff B, Motz W, Frenzel H et al. Structural and functional alterations of the intramyocardial coronary arterioles in patients with arterial hypertension. Circulation 1993; 88: 993–1003.
20. Lip GY, Blann AD, Jones AF et al. Relation of endothelium, thrombogenesis, and hemorheology in systemic hypertension to ethnicity and left ventricular hypertrophy. Am J Cardiol 1997; 80: 1566.

21. Bader M. Role of the local renin–angiotensin system in cardiac damage: a minireview focusing on transgenic animal models. J Mol Cell Cardiol 2002; 34: 1455–62.
22. Dong Y, Wang X, Zhu H et al. Endothelin-1 gene and progression of blood pressure and left ventricular mass: longitudinal findings in youth. Hypertension 2004; 44: 884–90.
23. MacCarthy PA, Grieve DA, Li J-M et al. Impaired endothelial cell regulation of ventricular relaxation in cardiac hypertrophy. Role of reactive oxygen species and NADPH oxidase. Circulation 2001; 104: 2967.
24. Frey N, Olson EN. Modulating cardiac hypertrophy by manipulating myocardial lipid metabolism? Circulation 2002; 105: 1152–4.
25. Jamshidi Y, Montgomery HE, Hense H-W et al. Peroxisome proliferators-activated receptor α gene regulates left ventricular growth in response to exercise and hypertension. Circulation 2000; 103: 226–30.
26. Kelly DP. Peroxisome proliferators-activated receptor α as a genetic determinant of cardiac hypertrophic growth. Culprit or innocent bystander? Circulation 2002; 105: 1025–27.
27. Barger PM, Brandt JM, Leone TC et al. Deactivation of peroxisome proliferator-activated receptor-α during cardiac hypertrophic growth. J Clin Invest 2000; 105: 1723–30.
28. Frey N, Katus HA, Olsen EN, Hill JA. Hypertrophy of the heart. A new therapeutic target? Circulation 2004; 109: 1580–9.
29. Asakawa M, Takano H, Nagai T et al. Peroxisome proliferator-activated receptor γ plays a critical role in the inhibition of cardiac hypertrophy in vitro and in vivo. Circulation 2002; 105: 1240–6.
30. Inzucchi SE. Oral antihyperglycemic therapy for type 2 diabetes. Scientific review. JAMA 2002; 287: 360–72.
31. Dawson A, Orrius AD, Struthers AD. The epidemiology of left ventricular hypertrophy in type 2 diabetes mellitus. Diabetologia 2005; 48: 1971–9.
32. Hill D, Millner D. Insulin as a growth factor. Pediatr Res 1985; 19: 879–86.
33. Adachi A, Ito H, Akimoto H et al. Insulin-like growth factor-II induces hypertrophy with increased expression of muscle-specific genes in cultured rat myocytes. J Mol Cell Cardiol 1994; 26: 789–95.
34. Sader S, Nian M, Liu P. Leptin. A novel link between obesity, diabetes, cardiovascular risk, and ventricular hypertrophy. Circulation 2003; 108: 644–6.
35. Barouch LA, Berkowitz DE, Harrison RW et al. Disruption of leptin signaling contributes to cardiac hypertrophy independently of body weight in mice. Circulation 2003; 108: 754–9.
36. Molkentin JD, Olsen EN. GATA-4: A novel transcriptional regulator of cardiac hypertrophy? Circulation 1997; 96: 3833–5.
37. Dimitrow PP, Galderisi M, Rigo F. The non-invasive documentation of coronary microcirculation impairment: role of transthoracic echocardiography. Cardiovasc Ultrasound 2005: 3: 18–26.
38. Kozàkovà M, de Simone G, Morizzo C, Palombo C. Coronary vasodilator capacity and hypertension-induced increase in left ventricular mass. Hypertension 2003; 41: 224.
39. Marcus ML, Koyanagi S, Harrison DG, et al. Abnormalities in the coronary circulation that occur as a consequence of cardiac hypertrophy. Am J Med 1983; 75: 62–6.
40. Palmieri V, Storto G, Arezzi E et al. Relations of left ventricular mass and systolic function to endocardial function and coronary flow reserve in healthy, new discovered hypertensive subjects. J Hum Hypertens 2005; 10: 1–10.
41. Gimelli A, Schneider-Eicke J, Neglia D et al. Homogeneously reduced versus regionally impaired myocardial blood flow in hypertensive patients: two different patterns of myocardial perfusion associated with the degree of hypertrophy. J Am Coll Cardiol 1998; 31: 366.
42. Roman MJ, Pickering TG, Schwartz JE et al. Relation of arterial structure and function to left ventricular geometric patterns in hypertensive adults. J Am Coll Cardiol 1996; 28: 751–6.
43. Strauer BE, Schwartzkopff B. Objectives of high blood pressure treatment: left ventricular hypertrophy, diastolic function, and coronary reserve. Am J Hypertens 1998; 11: 879–81.
44. Kataoka T, Hamasaki S, Ishida S et al. Contribution of increased minimal coronary resistance and attenuated vascular adaptive remodeling to myocardial ischemia in patients with systemic hypertension and ventricular hypertrophy. Am J Cardiol 2004; 94: 484–7.

45. Laine H, Katoh C, Luotolahti M et al. Myocardial oxygen consumption is unchanged but efficiency is reduced in patients with essential hypertension and left ventricular hypertrophy. Circulation 1999; 100: 2425.
46. Heidland UE, Strauer BE. Left ventricular muscle mass and elevated heart rate are associated with coronary plaque disruption. Circulation 2001; 104: 1477–82.
47. Roman MJ, Pickering TG, Schwartz JE, Pini R, Devereux RB. Relation of blood pressure variability to carotid atherosclerosis and carotid artery and left ventricular hypertrophy. Arterioscler Thromb Vasc Biol 2001; 21: 1507–11.
48. Roman MJ, Devereux RB, Schwartz JE et al. Arterial stiffness in chronic inflammatory diseases. Hypertension 2005; 46: 194–9.
49. Yildiz A, Memisoglu E, Oflaz H et al. Atherosclerosis and vascular calcification are independent predictors of left ventricular hypertrophy in chronic hemodialysis patients. Nephrol Dial Transplant 2005; 20: 760–7.
50. Chen CH, Ting CT, Lin, SJ et al. Which arterial and cardiac parameters best predict left ventricular mass? Circulation 1998; 98: 422–8.
51. Safar ME, Levy BI, Struijker-Boudier H. Current perspectives on arterial stiffness and pulse pressure in hypertension and cardiovascular diseases. Circulation 2003; 107: 2864–9.

2

Ultrasound contrast-enhanced stress echocardiography

Attila Nemes, Marcel L Geleijnse,
Osama II Soliman, Boudewijn J Krenning,
Willem B Vletter, and Folkert J ten Cate

Two-dimensional (2D) stress echocardiography is a non-invasive stress modality with a continuously evolving spectrum of indications. One of the most important indications is the identification of patients with coronary artery disease (CAD). For this purpose, wall motion of left ventricular (LV) segments is compared between rest, low-dose, and peak stress on several standardized LV views. The rationale for the use of 2D stress echocardiography is that cardiovascular stress will, in the presence of significant coronary artery disease, result in myocardial ischemia, manifested as a regional wall motion abnormality. Several methods (exercise, pharmacologic-induced, others) can be used during stress echocardiography. One of the most frequently used methods is dobutamine stress echocardiography. This method has a high sensitivity, specificity, and accuracy for CAD, including information on extent, severity, and localization of significant stenoses.[1]

Although the diagnostic and prognostic role of 2D stress echocardiography is well established, it is widely known that stress echocardiography suffers from a number of limitations. Suboptimal diagnostic accuracy may be caused by inadequate image quality, comparisons of non-identical LV wall segments at rest, low-dose, and peak stress, and smaller ischemic areas may be missed in the limited available LV cross-sections. Also, interpretation of 2D stress echocardiography is subjective, with different existing definitions of abnormality and considerable interobserver and interinstitutional diagnostic variability.[2] Ultrasound contrast agents have been successfully applied during 2D dobutamine stress echocardiography to improve endocardial border delineation. The use of intravenous ultrasound contrast improves endocardial border visualization, leading to a more accurate interpretation of wall motion abnormalities (Figure 2.1).[3]

Three-dimensional (3D) stress echocardiography has been advocated to improve the suboptimal diagnostic accuracy.[4] This has been available for several years, using time-consuming reconstruction techniques. However, recent advances in transducer technology and front-end data processing have brought real-time 3D echocardiography (RT3DE) into clinical practice. RT3DE has several advantages over conventional 2D echocardiographic methods. While 2D echocardiography makes incorrect geometric assumptions about LV morphology, 3D echocardiography sees the LV as it truly is. RT3DE is easy to learn and

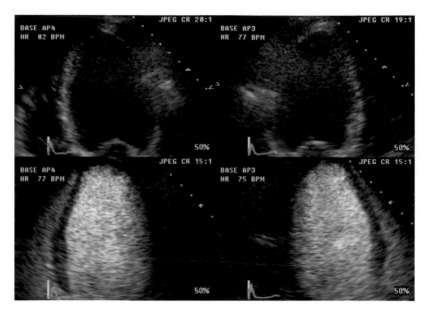

Figure 2.1 Stress 2D echocardiographic images with (lower images) and without (upper images) contrast agent.

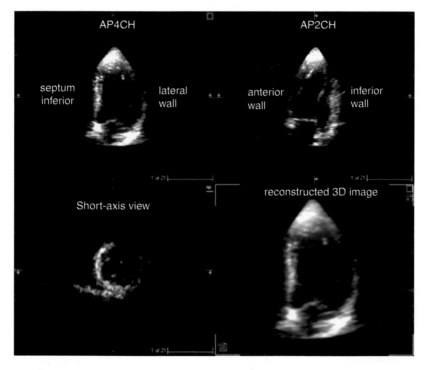

Figure 2.2 Automatically cropped images during real-time 3D echocardiography (without contrast agent). Abbreviations: AP4CH: apical 4-chamber view, AP2CH: apical 2-chamber view.

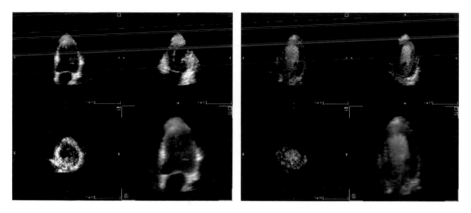

Figure 2.3 The use of ultrasound contrast agent improves the endocardial border detection during stress real-time 3D echocardiography (left: without contrast, right: with contrast). Order of images as in Figure 2.2.

is a less time-consuming imaging modality. As pointed out earlier, RT3DE has excellent correlation with cardiac magnetic resonance imaging for evaluation of LV volume, mass, and ejection fraction with comparable reproducibility. With stress RT3DE, at each stress level only one 3D data acquisition from one window is needed instead of multiple 2D data acquisitions from multiple windows (Figures 2.2 and 2.3). This makes a 3D examination faster than conventional 2D stress imaging. RT3DE allows analysis of similar segments in more detail from different planes simply by cropping and rotating the 3D volumetric data set, helping the identification of small ischemic LV regions. RT3DE allows anyplane evaluation of the LV, helping to create short-axis views at different LV levels that may be easier to understand by other (non-cardiologist) physicians.

Notwithstanding its great opportunities, at this moment stress RT3DE has a number of technical limitations. The primary restriction for RT3DE is the limited spatial volume coverage, or actually the trade-off between spatial volume, spatial resolution, and temporal resolution (3D frame rate). Visualization of the LV anterior wall can sometimes be difficult even during 2D echocardiography. Unfortunately, the anterior wall is inadequately visualized in a considerable number of our stress 3D examinations.[5] These problems are related to the relatively large footprint of the X4 matrix transducer compared to a standard S3 transducer (24×20 vs 24×15 mm), leading to rib shadowing. Currently, a transducer with a smaller footprint is available with the Philips iE33, which will result in better images.

Myocardial contrast echocardiography (MCE) is a non-invasive technique able to assess myocardial function and perfusion.[6] Recent studies have confirmed the ability of MCE to predict the improvement of myocardial function after reperfusion in acute myocardial infarction. The basis of this method is that after recording the baseline images, myocardial perfusion images can be obtained during contrast injection in real time (power modulation) using a low mechanical index (0.1). A slow bolus of 0.75 ml of sulfur hexafluoride (Sonovue, Bracco, Italy) can be intravenously injected, followed by a slow saline flush (5 ml)

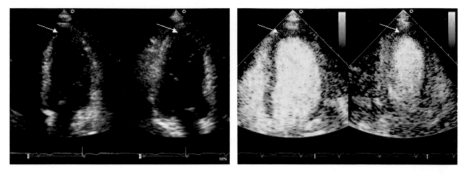

Figure 2.4   Myocardial contrast echocardiography can help in the identification of infarcted area. Left: without contrast, arrow: infarcted area at the apex of left ventricle; right: perfusion echo, arrow: in the infarcted area there is no perfusion indicating scar or no reflow.

for 5 seconds. Also Optison (sonicated albumin with perfluoropropane as a gas) is widely used for this purpose. If LV opacification and myocardial perfusion are not optimal, additional doses of 0.5 ml of contrast agent can be injected. Real-time power modulation imaging begins before contrast injection, and 'flash' imaging with a high mechanical index (1.6) is used at peak contrast intensity to destroy the microbubbles in the myocardium to exclude artifacts and to visualize myocardial contrast replenishment (15 cycles). After the real-time perfusion study, LV opacification images for endocardial border assessment are recorded using a 0.4 mechanical index to improve quantitative assessment of regional and global myocardial function (Figure 2.4).

These findings might indicate that both 2D and 3D stress echocardiography are suitable methods for the detection of CAD. However, the use of ultrasound contrast agents is necessary to improve the image quality. Myocardial contrast echocardiography may contribute to the identification of infarcted area or perfusion abnormalities.

REFERENCES

1. Geleijnse ML, Fioretti PM, Roelandt JR. Methodology, feasibility, safety and diagnostic accuracy of dobutamine stress echocardiography. J Am Coll Cardiol 1997; 30(3): 595–606.
2. Picano E, Lattanzi F, Orlandini A et al. Stress echocardiography and the human factor: the importance of being expert. J Am Coll Cardiol 1991; 17: 666–9.
3. Kasprzak JD, Paelinck B, Ten Cate FJ et al. Comparison of native and contrast-enhanced harmonic echocardiography for visualization of left ventricular endocardial border. Am J Cardiol 1999; 83: 211–17.
4. Franke A, Kuhl HP. Second-generation real-time 3D echocardiography: a revolutionary new technology, MedicaMundi 2003; 47: 34–40.
5. Nemes A, Geleijnse ML, Krenning BJ et al. Usefulness of ultrasound contrast agent to improve image quality during real-time three-dimensional stress echocardiography. Am J Cardiol 2007; 99: 275–8.
6. Biagini E, van Geuns RJ, Baks T et al. Comparison between contrast echocardiography and magnetic resonance imaging to predict improvement of myocardial function after primary coronary intervention. Am J Cardiol 2006; 97: 361–6.

3

Measurement of coronary artery flow by transthoracic Doppler ultrasound

Paolo Voci and Francesco Pizzuto

Which role for the microcirculation? • **Coronary artery disease**
• **A companion to computed tomography** • **Conclusion**

Coronary angiography, obtained either invasively or more recently non-invasively, shows the anatomic printout of the coronary arteries, but provides little information on the function of the arterial conduit, which is an important parameter for clinical decision-making, particularly in intermediate coronary lesions. Transthoracic coronary Doppler ultrasound is a recently developed extension of echocardiography,[1-9] which allows direct measurement of coronary flow velocity at the patient's bedside, thus providing non-invasively the functional information missed at coronary angiography.

Our knowledge on coronary flow velocity and coronary flow reserve (CFR) derives from the seminal observations by Lance Gould and his coworkers,[10-14] who described in animals and over 30 years ago the basics of coronary flow physiology that we still use in our daily clinical practice using transthoracic Doppler ultrasound. Lance Gould described CFR as a very simple measure obtained from the ratio between hyperemic and baseline flow (Figure 3.1). CFR basically describes the amount of coronary blood flow that we can spend at stress: in normal young subjects CFR may range between 3 and 6, which means that our coronary circulation is able to increase flow up to 6 times from resting values to meet the metabolic demand at stress. CFR is not only a simple, but also a quantitative and repeatable measure, that is characterized by a low intra- and interobserver variability,[14] and despite the fact that it can be measured only in a small tract of a coronary artery, it provides a number of clinically relevant information.

Other important experimental findings by Gould and coworkers, that were later confirmed in humans, are that:

(1) a coronary stenosis does not significantly impair flow at rest, and
(2) hyperemic flow is preserved until the stenosis reaches the critical value of 60-70%.

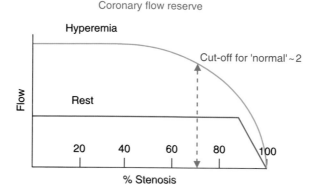

Figure 3.1   The classical curve by Lance Gould and coworkers[10] describing the relation between the degree of a coronary stenosis, artificially produced in dogs by coronary artery ligation, and coronary flow reserve (CFR). CFR is calculated as the ratio between hyperemic and baseline flow. The cut-off value of 2 discriminates significant (≥70%) from non-significant coronary stenosis. (Modified from reference 10.)

Beyond this point, CFR drops below the critical point of 2, a commonly accepted cut-off value discriminating a significant from a non-significant coronary lesion. Progressive restriction of the coronary artery further reduces CFR to the point that, when the artery is subocccluded, the hyperemic response disappears, which means that CFR drops to around or below 1 (Figure 3.1).

Maximal hyperemic flow can be easily elicited by venous infusion of natural compounds (ATP, or its byproduct adenosine) which are pure and potent coronary microvascular dilators having little or no effect on the diameter of the epicardial artery.[15,16] These characteristics are essential for correct measurement of CFR by ultrasound. Coronary flow is in fact the product of velocity times the cross-sectional area of the vessel, and because the diameter of the epicardial artery remains constant during adenosine infusion,[15,16] velocity can be used as a surrogate measure of flow. Adenosine is more commercially available than ATP. It is found in variable concentrations in human tissues, and can be safely used either in outpatients or in critically-ill patients, such as those with severe multivessel coronary artery disease (CAD) and acute myocardial infarction (AMI),[17] if employed appropriately. An infusion of 140 μg/kg/min for 90 seconds is sufficient to elicit maximal hyperemia, and most importantly it is safe, because hyperemia is so transient that the development of ischemia is prevented. Low-dose bolus injection (6 mg in 10–15 seconds) is also effective, safe, and cheap (20 dollars or less). Compared to other non-invasive imaging modalities, transthoracic coronary Doppler is a fast, flexible, repeatable, radiation-free, and real-time procedure requiring few cardiac cycles for measurement of CFR.

WHICH ROLE FOR THE MICROCIRCULATION?

CFR describes the cumulative effect on coronary flow of the epicardial coronary stenosis and the vasodilator capacity of the microcirculation. A microvascular dysfunction has been hypothesized in many clinical settings and in several systemic diseases, particularly in hypertension and diabetes. If the microcirculation were a prominent factor affecting CFR, there would be too many confounding factors preventing a reliable clinical use of CFR dysfunction to detect an epicardial stenosis. In fact, the interaction between microcirculation disease/dysfunction and CFR is not at all clear, and after a 10-year daily experience with transthoracic coronary Doppler ultrasound we may conclude that the role of microcirculation has been overemphasized in the medical literature. This position is demonstrated by the following clinical examples:

(1) Coronary stenting was believed to produce a microvascular dysfunction lasting for days or weeks,[18-20] but we have challenged this concept, showing that CFR rapidly normalizes after the procedure (Figure 3.2).[14]
(2) Focal coronary artery disease was supposed to generate a diffuse alteration in coronary flow, involving not only the stenosed artery, but also angiographically normal (remote) coronary arteries[21] in a generalized, but still unexplained, derangement of microvascular flow. Conversely, we have found that CFR in the angiographically normal coronary artery is never affected by any remote stenosis, previous AMI, or stenting (Figure 3.3).[22] Therefore focal factors in each territory are the major determinants of CFR in patients with CAD, and impaired CFR in one region is not a general

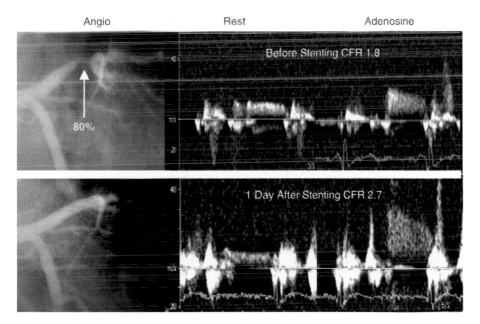

Figure 3.2 Coronary flow reserve (CFR) normalizes early after coronary stenting, demonstrating that the microcirculation has little or no influence at all in this setting.

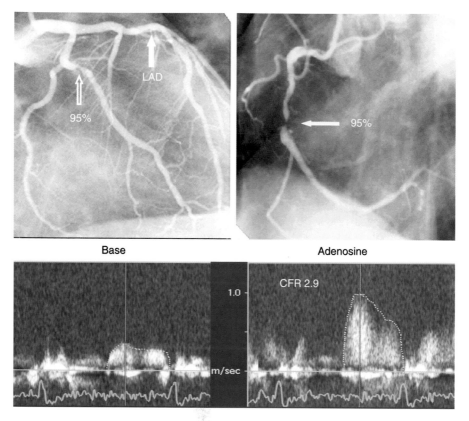

Figure 3.3 Upper panels: coronary angiography of a patient with angiographically normal left anterior descending coronary artery (LAD) and remote significant coronary stenosis shows a 95% stenosis of the first obtuse marginal branch (open arrow on the left panel) and a 90% stenosis of the middle tract (solid arrow on the right panel) of the right coronary artery. Lower panels: coronary flow reserve (CFR) of the LAD, measured by transthoracic Doppler ultrasound, shows a value of 2.9, within the range of the control group. (Reproduced from reference 22.)

phenomenon of the coronary circulation. Similarly,[15] serial assessments along the coronary artery by intracoronary Doppler ultrasound invariably show that CFR is impaired only distal to the stenosis, but not proximal to it (Figure 3.4).

(3) Microvascular involvement is often called to explain cyclic chest pain and positive stress tests in fertile women with normal epicardial coronary arteries, but a confirmation of this link is lacking.[23-28] In fact, only minor changes in CFR are found in association with varying hormonal exposure, which certainly cannot explain positive stress tests.[29]

(4) Active and passive cigarette smoke may alter coronary vasomotion and microvascular flow, but the relative changes in CFR are again minor,[30] and well above the threshold value of 2.24[31]–2.5[32] accepted for significant

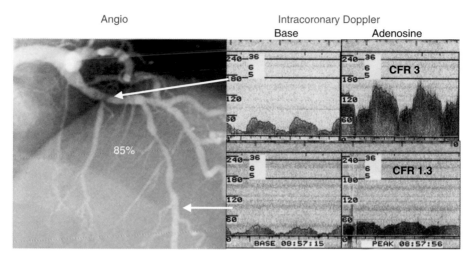

Figure 3.4   Intracoronary Doppler ultrasound during intracoronary bolus injection of adenosine (36 μg). CFR is normal proximal to the coronary stenosis, whereas it is markedly impaired distal to it, confirming the pivotal role of the stenosis, compared to the microcirculation. (Reproduced from reference 15.)

microvascular dysfunction. Similarly, studies using positron emission tomography showed no difference in CFR between smokers and non smokers.[33]

In our daily practice with transthoracic coronary Doppler ultrasound, we have found that pure microvascular dysfunction resulting in CFR < 2 is a rare exception, not only in patients with non-insulin-dependent diabetes mellitus and hypertension (Figure 3.5), but even in patients with serious diseases such as dilated (Figure 3.6) or hypertrophic (Figure 3.7) cardiomyopathies. These findings reinforce the use of transthoracic Doppler ultrasound to detect epicardial CAD independently from the effects of microcirculation in a wide range of cardiac diseases, including hypertension and diabetes, where other imaging modalities, including very expensive tools such as positron emission tomography, have shown dependency.

CORONARY ARTERY DISEASE

Coronary stenosis

A flow-limiting stenosis introduces a strong proximal resistance that is higher than that opposed by the microcirculation, as demonstrated by the early normalization of CFR after the mechanical relief of the stenosis by coronary stenting (Figure 3.2).[14]

Several authors using single photon emission computed tomography,[34,35] intracoronary,[36] and transthoracic coronary Doppler ultrasound[3–8,37–39] have adopted the Gould's 'magic number' of 2 as the cut-off value discriminating significant

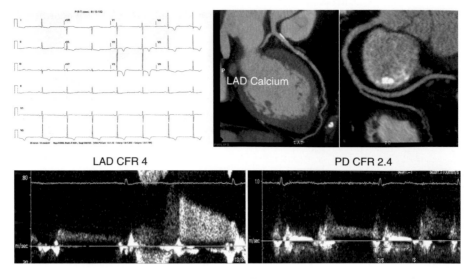

Figure 3.5 Hypertensive patient with resting diffuse T-wave inversion. Computed tomography was non-diagnostic because of coronary calcifications, whereas CFR was normal in both the LAD and in the posterior descending coronary artery (PD).

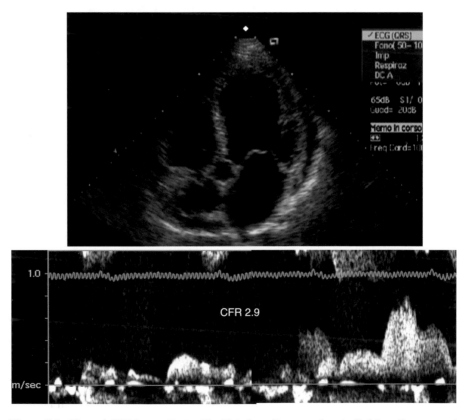

Figure 3.6 Normal CFR in a patient with dilated cardiomyopathy studied in orthopnea and showing pericardial and pleural effusion.

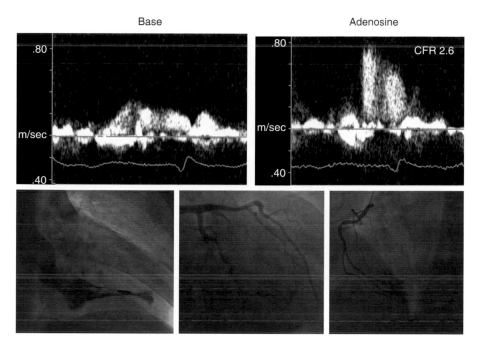

Figure 3.7 Normal CFR in a patient with hypertrophic cardiomyopathy.

impairment of coronary flow that should be treated invasively. In clinical practice, transthoracic coronary Doppler ultrasound may be a quantitative and repeatable measure to monitor patients and to help defer revascularization in those having a CFR above 2,[40] with important economic, ethical, and social implications, particularly in the light of our recent concern about the excess of unnecessary invasive treatment in patients with CAD.

In keeping with the experimental findings,[10,11] transthoracic coronary Doppler ultrasound correlates well with the angiographic degree of the stenosis (Figure 3.8).[8,14,37] This is true for non-significant (< 50%) and significant (≥70%) coronary lesions, but data on intermediate (50–69%) lesions[41-43] are more dispersed (Figure 3.9). This is not surprising, since intermediate lesions are difficult to quantify, even with quantitative coronary angiography.[44]

Coronary subocclusion

We have learned from the Coronary Artery Surgery Study registry that patients with >90% stenosis have a 7.5 times higher probability of developing acute myocardial infarction than those with less severe lesions.[45] Therefore, it appears to be important to discriminate patients with coronary subocclusion from those with less important lesions. Transthoracic coronary Doppler ultrasound can

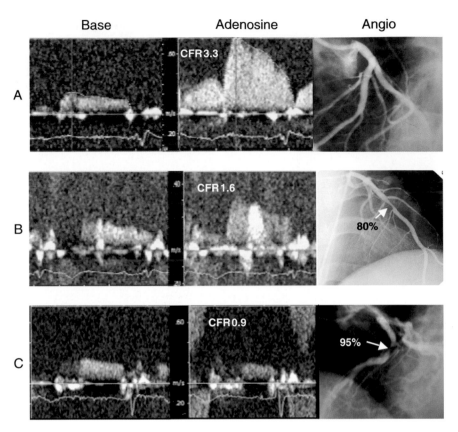

Figure 3.8 Non-invasive measurement of CFR by Doppler echocardiography compared to coronary angiography in patients with normal (A), significant (B), and severe (C) left anterior descending CAD. Severe disease is characterized by damped flow reserve. (Reproduced from reference 43.)

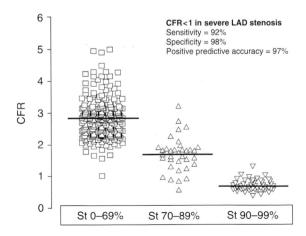

Figure 3.9 Peak diastolic CFR in the three groups of patients with left anterior descending CAD shows damped CFR in patients with >90% stenosis. (Reproduced from reference 43.)

detect subocclusion, because the hyperemic response disappears at >90% vessel stenosis (Figures 3.8, 3.9 and 3.10).[14,43] Several mechanisms may be called to explain this phenomenon:

(1) In very tight stenoses, the microvascular vasodilator reserve may be already exhausted at rest and cannot increase any further under stress.
(2) An incompletely calcified coronary stenosis may collapse during adenosine infusion[12,13,44] for a Venturi effect.[44]
(3) Prestenotic collaterals may open under stress, stealing blood from the ischemic territory to perfuse remote, less jeopardized segments (Figure 3.11).[45]

A relative increase in systolic coronary flow velocity at rest has also been proposed as a marker of severe stenosis,[46] but further studies are needed to confirm the diagnostic value of this parameter, which has the important potential advantage of being obtained by a simple resting exam.

Coronary occlusion

Reverse diastolic flow at rest reflects retrograde filling of the artery by collaterals, and is a very specific marker of coronary occlusion[47] (Figure 3.12). However, collaterals may perfuse the vessel not only retrogradely but also anterogradely

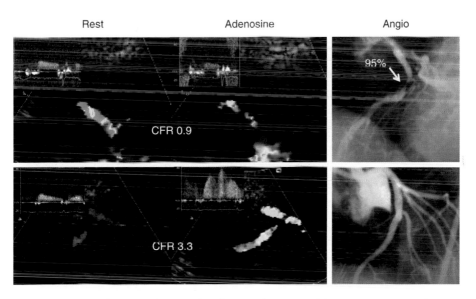

Figure 3.10 Transthoracic color Doppler ultrasound imaging of the LAD. Upper panels show decreased signal intensity with color Doppler imaging and damped (0.9) CFR with pulsed wave Doppler ultrasound in a patient with severe LAD stenosis, providing an online detection of coronary steal. Lower panels show, for comparison, the increase in signal intensity with color Doppler imaging and a normal (3.3) CFR with pulsed wave Doppler ultrasound in a patient with non-significant LAD disease. (Reproduced from reference 43.)

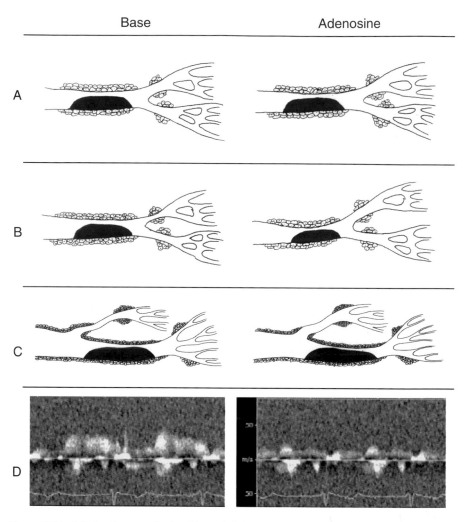

Figure 3.11   Mechanisms producing blunted flow reserve in severe coronary artery stenosis. (A) Maximal resting microvascular dilation due to a too tight stenosis; (B) stenosis collapse; (C) coronary steal; (D) transthoracic coronary Doppler ultrasound shows reduced coronary flow velocity during adenosine infusion. See text for details. (Reproduced from reference 43.)

in up to 50% of cases,[48–50] therefore the finding of retrograde flow has high specificity but low sensitivity in detecting coronary occlusion. The response of collateral flow to vasodilator stress can be measured by transthoracic Doppler ultrasound (Figures 3.13 and 3.14).[48] It may add useful prognostic information on the functional impact of the collateral circulation, and in the future may be a useful non-invasive measure to monitor the efficacy of innovative perfusion therapies as neoangiogenesis.

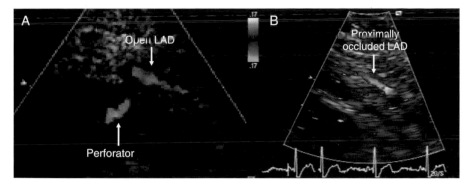

Figure 3.12   (A) Color flow Doppler ultrasound of a subject with normal anterograde flow both in the distal LAD, coded in blue, and in a perforator, coded in red. (B) Patient with occluded LAD and inverted flow in the distal tract of the artery, coded in blue at color Doppler ultrasound. (Reproduced from reference 48.)

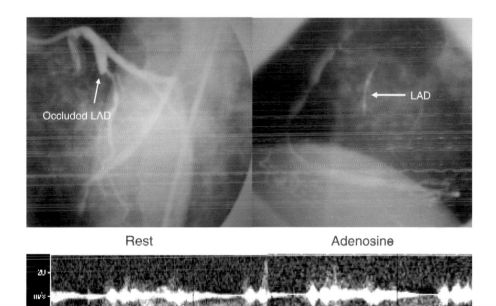

Figure 3.13   Upper panels: coronary angiography of a patient with proximally occluded LAD and poor (Rentrop grade 1) collaterals from the right coronary artery. Lower panels: flow in the LAD measured by transthoracic Doppler ultrasound is retrograde, and CFR is 0.8. (Reproduced from reference 48.)

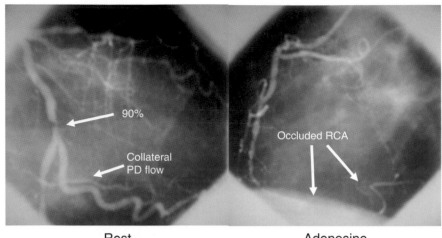

Rest   Adenosine

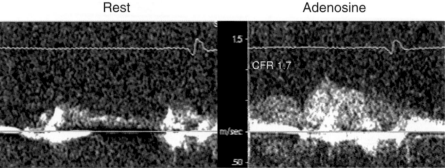

Figure 3.14   Upper panels: coronary angiography of a patient with occlusion of the distal tract of the right coronary artery (RCA). The collateral flow feeding the PD and posterolateral coronary arteries (Rentrop grade 3) is supplied by the proximal portion of the RCA and by septal branches of the LAD (a combination of anterograde and retrograde collateral flows, supplied by multiple sources of collaterals). The patient also had a tight stenosis of the circumflex coronary artery (arrow). Lower panels: the CFR, assessed by transthoracic Doppler ultrasound in the PD, is 1.7. (Reproduced from reference 48.)

Coronary stenting

The implantation of a coronary artery stent modifies the anatomy and pathophysiology of the treated coronary segment and stabilizes the atherosclerotic plaque. According to these changes in the coronary arterial wall morphology and reactivity, patients with stents often have atypical symptoms, and their responses to the standard non-invasive diagnostic tests may be inconclusive, particularly in single-vessel disease. Over a number of years we have followed our patients with LAD stents with serial measurements, and we have found that a CFR <2 identifies a ≥70% LAD in-stent restenosis,[51,52] whereas a CFR between 2 and 2.5 reflects a non-significant (intermediate) in-stent restenosis, that should be conservatively monitored, whilst treatment can safely be deferred when the CFR is above 2 (Figures 3.15 and 3.16).[40] Other authors[38,53] have utilized resting flow acceleration at the percutaneous transluminal coronary angioplasty (PTCA) stent site to predict restenosis. Unfortunately, the technology is not ready to allow complete scanning of the LAD, but undoubtedly the ability to detect a coronary gradient at rest along a coronary artery[54] (Figure 3.17) is a fascinating research area requiring extensive investment in ultrasound technology.

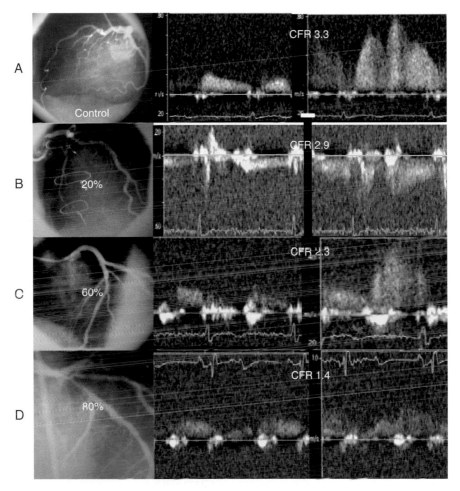

Figure 3.15   (A) Transthoracic resting and hyperemic Doppler velocities of a patient with a CFR of 3.3 and corresponding coronary angiography, showing a normal LAD. (B) Patient with LAD stent implanted 66 months before. At follow-up, CFR was 2.9 and corresponding angiography showed a 20% in-stent narrowing. (C) Patient with a non-invasive CFR of 2.3 and corresponding coronary angiography, showing focal 60% middle LAD in-stent restenosis. (D) A patient with a non-invasive CFR of 1.4 and the corresponding angiography, showing diffuse 80% middle LAD in-stent restenosis. (Reproduced from reference 52.)

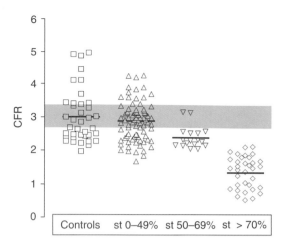

Figure 3.16 CFR is shown individually in control subjects and patients with LAD stents and different degrees of in-stent restenosis. Confidence intervals (99%) of the average value obtained in control subjects are shown in shaded form to provide a direct comparison to visually estimate how the two parameters distribute according to the groups considered. Thick lines represent average values in each subgroup. Of note, only one individual with ≥50% in-stent restenosis had a CFR lying in the confidence intervals of controls, whereas most of those with ≥70% in-stent restenosis had values < 2 (Reproduced from reference 52.)

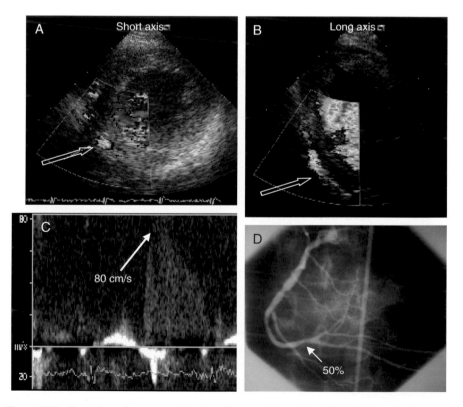

Figure 3.17 Transthoracic coronary Doppler ultrasound scanning of the PD shows an inappropriate acceleration at the level of the crux cordis (arrows), which corresponds to a 50% stenosis at coronary angiography. (Reproduced from reference 54.)

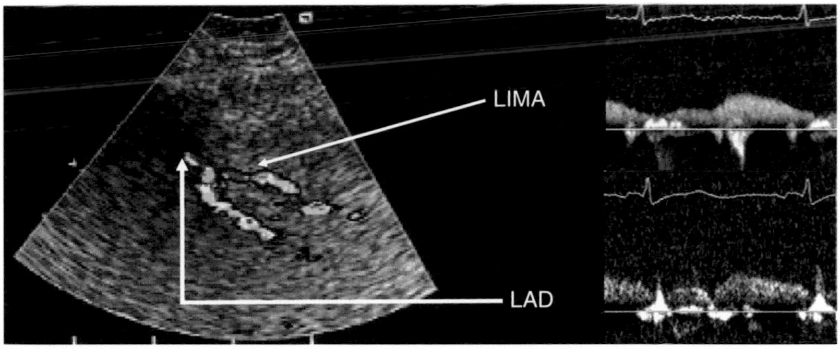

LIMA Graft

Figure 3.18   Transthoracic coronary Doppler ultrasound imaging of the left internal mammary artery to the LAD graft and corresponding pulsed Doppler tracings. (Reproduced from reference 59.)

Coronary grafts

It is very easy to measure flow in the left and right internal mammary arteries both at the origin[55-57] and at the level of the suture over the LAD (Figure 3.18).[1,2,58,59] For saphenous vein grafts, flow can be measured mainly at the level of the suture over the LAD. Imaging of grafts to other coronary arteries definitely depends on further improvements in ultrasound technology. Coronary Doppler ultrasound adds new information on the pathophysiology of flow in the graft-to-coronary conduit. We have recently shown that measuring CFR in the graft alone may underestimate the functional capacity of the conduit. In fact, flow competition from a non-occluded recipient artery may reduce flow in the graft despite its full patency (Figure 3.19). CFR should therefore be measured in the distal tract of the recipient artery, which is not affected by flow competition and best reflects the patency status of the arterial conduit.[59]

Obtaining more arteries

Despite the prominence of the LAD in the prognosis of CAD, the evaluation of other coronary arteries is also desirable. As most of the infarctions occur either in the LAD or in the PD distribution territories,[60] we have recently concentrated on PD flow (Figure 3.20).[42] In our experience, it is feasible to measure CFR in the LAD in around 98% of patients, but unfortunately the feasibility drops to around 50% for the PD.[42] The PD is difficult to image for anatomic and technical reasons:

(1) It runs deep into the chest whereas the LAD is more superficial.
(2) It runs close to the right ventricular inflow tract and to the mid cardiac vein, which generate strong and disturbing flow signals (Figure 3.21).[42]
(3) Adenosine-induced hyperventilation interferes more with PD than with LAD imaging.
(4) For the LAD, but not for the PD, a dedicated transducer has been designed.

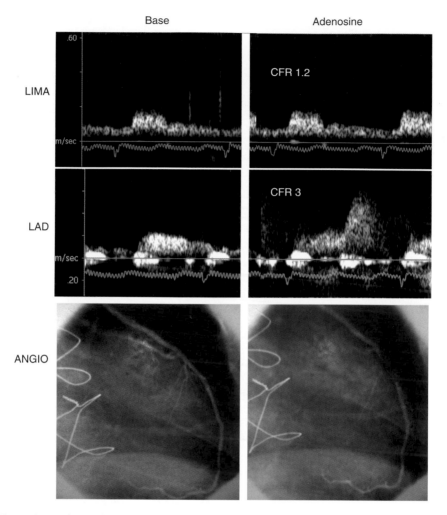

Figure 3.19 Flow competition between the internal mammary artery (LIMA) and the LAD. Upper panels: flow velocity in the LIMA shows a higher systolic than diastolic component, and a markedly abnormal CFR. Middle panels: CFR, measured in the distal LAD, is normal. Lower panels: coronary angiography shows that the LIMA is proximally patent, but contrast material stopped at the joining tract, due to flow competition with the native vessel. (Reproduced from reference 59.)

Imaging of the PD can be improved in several ways, by:

- the use of ultrasound contrast agents;
- the use of specific A_{2A} adenosine receptor agonists or drug combinations reducing hyperventilation;[61]
- the design of specific probes and software; and
- reducing the heart rate to below 60 beats/min, to minimize wall motion artifacts on Doppler sampling.

Studies on these aspects are underway in our laboratory, and promise to improve PD imaging by up to 80%.

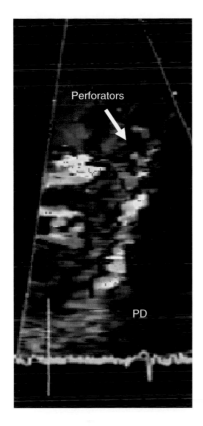

Figure 3.20 Transthoracic color Doppler echocardiography showing the PD and three perforating branches (arrow) at the level of the posterior papillary muscle.

Posterior Interventricular Groove Vessels

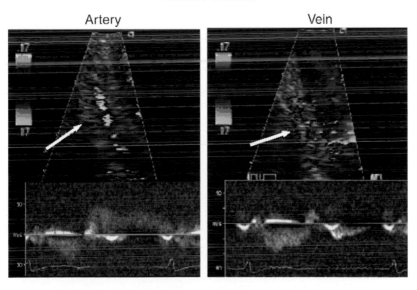

Figure 3.21 Transthoracic color Doppler imaging of the coronary vessels running in the posterior interventricular groove. The PD is characterized by an anterograde decrescendo diastolic flow coded in red, often with some aliasing (left panel), whereas the middle cardiac vein is characterized by a retrograde flow, coded in blue (right panel). (Reproduced from reference 42.)

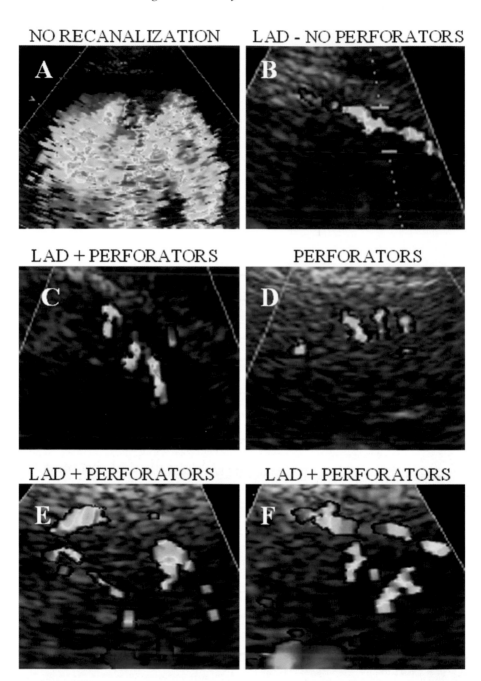

Figure 3.22 Different levels of recanalization, as assessed by high-resolution transthoracic color Doppler echocardiography after anterior myocardial infarction, help detecting reopening of the coronary artery and effective myocardial reperfusion. (A) Neither the LAD nor the perforators are imaged, in a patient with failed reperfusion and occluded LAD at angiography. (B) Patent LAD without perforating branches. (C and D) Imaging of perforating branches (non full-thickness recanalization). (E, F) Full thickness recanalization. (Reproduced from reference 62.)

Acute coronary syndromes

Detection of LAD patency before and after thrombolysis for AMI is a key feature of transthoracic Doppler echocardiography, and detection of perforators is a marker of effective, intramural recanalization after thrombolysis or percutaneous coronary interventions (Figure 3.22)[62] predicting recovery of left ventricular function at follow-up. Perforators bridge the large epicardial artery and the microcirculation, and their patency in AMI may yield the same information as myocardial contrast echocardiography[63] about the status of local nutrient perfusion.

Diastolic coronary flow velocity at rest may predict thronbolysis in myocardial infarction (TIMI) flow.[62] In fact, both Doppler ultrasound and TIMI flow measure velocities. However, the correlation between TIMI flow and Doppler ultrasound is imperfect (Figure 3.23), probably because the former is a semiquantitative and

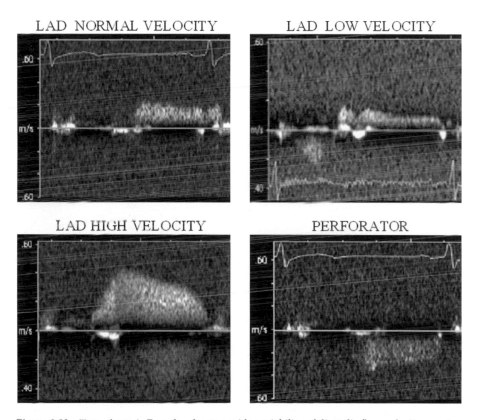

Figure 3.23   Transthoracic Doppler shows a wide variability of diastolic flow velocity, ranging from 15 to 40 cm/s, and of diastolic slope, regardless of effective revascularization. Left lower panel shows the distinctive, retrograde diastolic flow in a perforating branch. (Reproduced from reference 62.)

subjective measure, whereas the latter may be altered by vasomotor tone, thrombosis, and drugs administered during AMI.

Adenosine can be safely used during AMI,[17] and CFR provides important additive information about the viability of the microcirculation. Intracoronary studies have shown that a CFR ≥ 1.6 in the infarct-related artery is a sensitive marker of myocardial viability, predicting recovery of regional LV function at follow-up (Figure 3.24).[63] Therefore an integrated morphologic and functional approach by transthoracic coronary Doppler ultrasound (recanalization of perforators and measurement of CFR) may be a key prospective tool for clinical decision-making and prognostic stratification in AMI.

Other resting pulsed Doppler parameters, such as reverse systolic flow[64] and short deceleration time,[65] were associated with no-reflow, but these signs are not specific (Figure 3.25);[66,67] they are prone to artifacts and at least need further clinical validation.[68]

Several studies have shown that the cavitation effect of ultrasound, which is greatly enhanced by ultrasound contrast agents containing microbubbles, facilitates clot lysis through an acceleration of the enzymatic activity of recombinant tissue plasminogen activator (rtPA).[68,69] In AMI, direct imaging of the occluded coronary artery may enhance thrombolysis and potentially transform an emerging imaging modality into a fascinating therapeutic tool.[70]

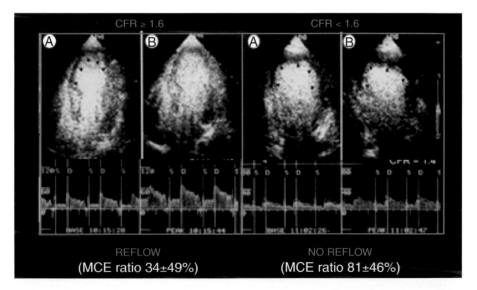

Figure 3.24 Intravenous myocardial contrast echocardiography (upper panels) and intracoronary Doppler ultrasound (lower panels) show that good reflow after acute anterior myocardial infarction parallels a good response in CFR. A cut-off value of CFR of 1.6 predicts good recovery of left ventricular function at follow-up, being a marker of adequate microcirculatory viability. (Reproduced from reference 63.)

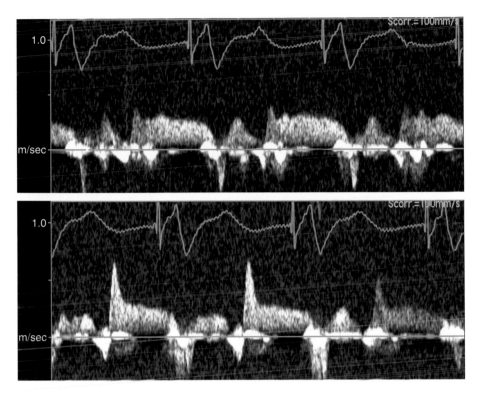

Figure 3.25 Patient with pacemaker rhythm. The LAD is first sampled on its central flow (upper panel) and then slightly angling the transducer laterally (lower panel). Artifacts due to probe positioning, muscle contraction and relaxation as well as venous flow may produce systolic and diastolic artifacts (lower panel) that should be distinguished from a true alteration of coronary flow velocity pattern. (Reproduced from reference 15.)

Comparison with other stress tests

Transthoracic coronary Doppler ultrasound has several advantages over other stress tests:

- It is accurate in detecting single vessel disease,[14,52] whereas exercise ECG, myocardial scintigraphy, and dobutamine echocardiography may not perform well.[71-73]
- It is low cost in terms of drug and personnel use.
- It is less time consuming, because only few baseline and hyperemic diastoles are needed to measure CFR.
- It provides a quantitative measure of coronary blood flow, which is particularly useful for follow-up evaluation.[52]
- It is independent of baseline ST alterations and bundle branch block (Figure 3.26).
- Drugs as beta-blockers and nitrates need not be discontinued.[74]
- It maintains its accuracy in diabetes, hypertension, and even in patients with previous homozonal myocardial infarction (unpublished data).

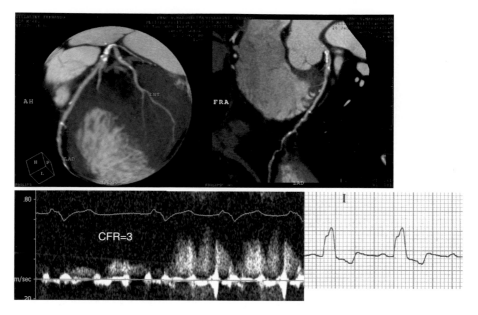

Figure 3.26   Multislice (40 rows) computed tomography of the coronary arteries in a patient with LAD stenting and left bundle branch block. Coronary calcium prevents evaluation of the coronary lumen, whereas transthoracic coronary Doppler ultrasound shows a good CFR. Coronary angiography confirms no luminal narrowing in the LAD.

A relative limitation of transthoracic coronary Doppler ultrasound is that, with the state-of-the-art technology, only the LAD can be studied with ease, whereas the PD is more difficult to detect, and there are no solid data on other arteries. However, we have to bear in mind that the LAD is the artery of life (or conversely the 'widow maker'), and that CFR in the LAD is an important predictor of cardiovascular events.[75,76]

Coronary vasomotion and the 'third dimension' of Doppler

Time and velocity are the most commonly used parameters to extrapolate clinically useful data from Doppler spectra. However, there is a third potentially useful but often neglected piece of information in the Doppler spectrum: the intensity of the reflected signal.[77] Provided that the entire section of the coronary artery is included in the sample volume, Doppler intensity is proportional to the number of scatterers and is a measure of blood volume crossing the Doppler sample volume. Doppler intensity can be used to detect coronary vasomotion: it may decrease during handgrip in patients with CAD when the sympathetic drive increases coronary vasomotor tone, whereas it may increase or remain unchanged in normals (Figure 3.27).[77] A similar response is observed during cigarette smoking[15] (Figure 3.28), when Doppler intensity may be more sensitive than CFR[30] in detecting subtle changes in coronary vasomotor tone.

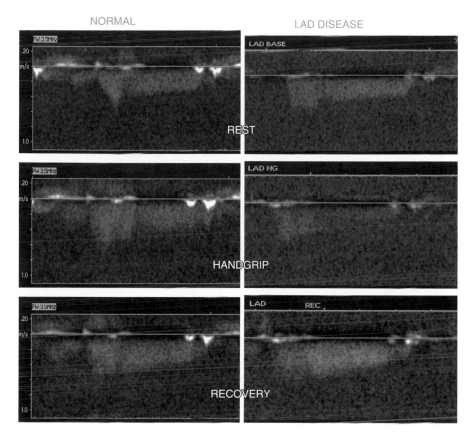

Figure 3.27 Coronary Doppler ultrasound tracing during 30 s handgrip. Left panels: in a subject with normal coronary arteries the intensity of the Doppler ultrasound signal remains unchanged throughout the test. Right panels: same test in a patient with significant LAD disease. The intensity of the Doppler ultrasound signal is reduced during handgrip, probably due to coronary vasoconstriction, and is slightly increased at recovery, probably due to reactive hyperemia. (Reproduced from reference 77.)

A COMPANION TO COMPUTED TOMOGRAPHY

Multislice computed tomography is a valuable technique to detect CAD. However, quantitation of a stenosis is difficult, and a non-negligible proportion of patients have coronary calcifications, motion artifacts, and/or arrhythmia that may prevent reliable measurement of the coronary lumen. In all these cases CFR may provide the functional data necessary to evaluate the physiologic impact of the underlying stenosis (Figure 3.26). On the other hand, computed tomography is very useful in imaging the early stages of atherosclerosis, and it may show pre-clinical lipid-rich plaques (Figure 3.29). CFR is an ideal complementary technique to assess the physiologic relevance of a stenosis, and may provide a useful

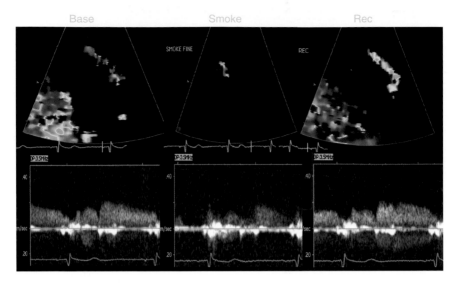

Figure 3.28 The effect of smoke on color Doppler ultrasound imaging and pulsed Doppler tracing. Coronary vasoconstriction caused by smoking is detected as a reduction in color Doppler flow signal, corresponding to a reduction in pulsed Doppler ultrasound intensity, which is followed by a recovery phase, characterized by some reactive hyperemia. (Reproduced from reference 15.)

Soft LAD plaque

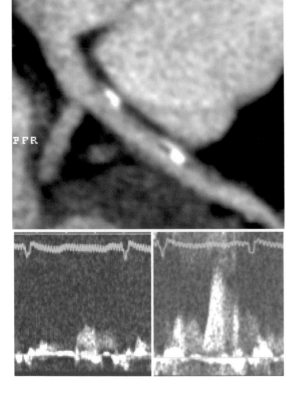

Figure 3.29 Multislice (40 rows) computed tomography of the coronary arteries in a patient with atypical symptoms and ECG stress interrupted for arrhythmias shows a non-significant fibro-lipidic plaque with small spots of calcification. Coronary flow reserve measured by transthoracic ultrasound is normal, and can be used for serial follow-up assessments, avoiding radiation exposure.

reference (baseline) value for serial follow-up assessments, without repeatedly exposing the patient to radiation.

CONCLUSION

Transthoracic coronary Doppler ultrasound is a valuable technique, providing a direct, not a surrogate, marker of coronary atherosclerosis.[78] Unfortunately, for some unexplained reason, it has not yet become popular, particularly in the US. No wonder, when Johan Christian Doppler announced to the scientific community of Konstanz the results of his observations on frequency shift, only six people, and probably all friends, came to listen to his funky results.

REFERENCES

1. Voci P, Testa G, Plaustro G et al. Assessment of coronary flow by high-resolution transthoracic echocardiography and non-directional Doppler ultrasound. Cardiologia 1997; 42(8): 849–53.
2. Voci P, Testa G, Plaustro G. Imaging of the distal left anterior descending coronary artery by transthoracic color-Doppler echocardiography. Am J Cardiol 1998; 81(12A): 74–8G.
3. Hozumi T, Yoshida K, Ogata Y et al. Noninvasive assessment of significant left anterior descending coronary artery stenosis by coronary flow velocity reserve with transthoracic color Doppler echocardiography. Circulation 1998; 97: 1557–62.
4. Hozumi T, Yoshida K, Akasaka T, et al. Noninvasive assessment of coronary flow velocity and coronary flow velocity reserve in the left anterior descending coronary artery by Doppler echocardiography. Comparison with invasive technique. J Am Coll Cardiol 1998; 32: 1251–9.
5. Caiati C, Montaldo C, Zedda N et al. New noninvasive method for coronary flow reserve assessment. Contrast-enhanced transthoracic second harmonic echo Doppler. Circulation 1999; 99: 771–8.
6. Caiati C, Zedda N, Montaldo C et al. Contrast enhanced transthoracic second harmonic echo Doppler with adenosine. A noninvasive, rapid and effective method for coronary flow reserve assessment. J Am Coll Cardiol 1999; 34: 122–30.
7. Caiati C, Montaldo C, Zedda N et al. Validation of a new noninvasive method (contrast-enhanced transthoracic second harmonic echo Doppler) for the evaluation of coronary flow reserve. Comparison with intracoronary Doppler flow wire. J Am Coll Cardiol 1999; 34: 1193–200.
8. Lambertz H, Tries HP, Stein T et al. Noninvasive assessment of coronary flow reserve with transthoracic signal-enhanced Doppler echocardiography. J Am Soc Echocardiogr 1999; 12: 186–95.
9. Daimon M, Watanabe H, Yamagishi H et al. Physiologic assessment of coronary artery stenosis by coronary flow reserve measurement with transthoracic Doppler echocardiography: comparison with exercise thallium-201 single photon emission computed tomography. J Am Coll Cardiol 2001; 37: 1310–15.
10. Gould KL, Lipscomb K. Effects of coronary stenoses on coronary flow reserve and resistance. Am J Cardiol 1974; 34: 48–55.
11. Gould KL, Lipscomb K, Hamilton GW. Physiologic basis for assessing severe coronary stenosis: instantaneous flow response and regional distribution during coronary hyperemia as measures of coronary flow reserve. Am J Cardiol 1974; 33: 87–94.
12. Gould KL. Dynamic coronary stenosis. Am J Cardiol 1980; 45: 286–92.
13. Gould KL. Collapsing coronary stenosis: a Starling resistor. Int J Cardiol 1982; 2: 39–42.
14. Pizzuto F, Voci P, Mariano E et al. Assessment of flow velocity reserve by transthoracic Doppler and venous adenosine infusion, before and after left anterior descending coronary stenting. J Am Coll Cardiol 2001; 38: 155–62.

15. Voci P, Pizzuto F, Romeo F. Coronary flow: a new asset for the echo lab? Eur Heart J 2004; 25: 1867–79.
16. Sudhir K, MacGregor JS, Barbant SD et al. Assesment of coronary conductance and resistance vessel reactivity in response to nitroglycerin, ergonovine and adenosine: in vivo studies with simultaneous intravascular two-dimensional and Doppler ultrasound. J Am Coll Cardiol 1993; 21: 1261–8.
17. Marzilli M, Orsini E, Marracini P, et al. Beneficial effects of intracoronary adenosine as an adjunct to primary angioplasty in acute myocardial infarction. Circulation 2000; 101: 2154–9
18. van Liebergen RAM, Piek JJ, Koch KT et al. Immediate and long term effect of balloon angioplasty or stent implantation on the absolute and relative coronary blood flow velocity reserve. Circulation 1998; 98: 2133–40.
19. Kern MJ, Puri S, Bach RG et al. Abnormal coronary flow velocity reserve after coronary artery stenting in patients. Role of relative coronary reserve to assess potential mechanisms. Circulation 1999; 100: 2491–8.
20. van Liebergen RAM, Piek JJ, Koch KT et al. Hyperemic coronary flow after optimized intravascular ultrasound-guided balloon angioplasty and stent implantation. J Am Coll Cardiol 1999; 34: 1899–906.
21. Uren NG, Crake T, Lefroy DC et al. Reduced coronary vasodilator function in infarcted and normal myocardium after myocardial infarction. N Engl J Med 1994; 331: 222–7.
22. Pizzuto F, Voci P, Mariano E et al. Coronary flow reserve of the angiographically normal left anterior descending coronary artery in patients with remote coronary artery disease. Am J Cardiol 2004; 94: 577–82.
23. Grodstein F, Stampfer MJ, Manson JE et al. Postmenopausal estrogen and progestin use and the risk of cardiovascular disease. N Engl J Med 1996; 335: 453–61.
24. Hu FB, Stampfer MJ, Manson JE et al. Trends in the incidence of coronary heart disease and changes in diet and lifestyle in women. N Engl J Med 2000; 343: 530
25. Herrington DM, Reboussin DM, Brosnihan B et al. Effects of estrogen replacement on the progression of coronary-artery atherosclerosis. N Engl J Med 2000; 343: 522–9.
26. Hsia J, Simon JA, Lin F et al. Peripheral arterial disease in randomized trial of estrogen with progestin in women with coronary heart disease. The Heart and Estrogen/Progestin Replacement study. Circulation 2000; 102: 2228–32.
27. Alexander KP, Newby LK, Hellkamp AS et al. Initiation of hormone replacement therapy after acute myocardial infarction is associated with more cardiac events during follow-up. J Am Coll Cardiol 2001; 38: 1–7.
28. Grady D, Hulley S B. Postmenopausal hormones and heart disease. J Am Coll Cardiol 2001; 38: 8–10.
29. Hirata K, Shimada K, Watanabe H et al. Modulation of coronary flow velocity reserve by sex, menstrual cycle and hormone replacement therapy. J Am Coll Cardiol 2001; 38: 1879–84.
30. Otsuka R, Watanabe H, Hirata K, et al. Acute effects of passive smoking on the coronary circulation in healthy young adults. JAMA 2001; 286: 436–41.
31. Bergmann SR, Herrero P, Markham P et al. Noninvasive quantification of myocardial blood flow in human subjects with ^{15}O-labeled water and positron emission tomography. J Am Coll Cardiol 1989; 14: 639–52.
32. Reis ES, Holubkov R, Lee JS et al. Coronary flow velocity response to adenosine characterizes coronary microvascular function in women with chest pain and no obstructive coronary disease: results from the pilot phase of Women's Ischemia Syndrome Evaluation (WISE) Study. J Am Coll Cardiol 1999; 33: 1469–75.
33. Campisi R, Czernin J, Schoeder H et al. Effect of long-term smoking on myocardial blood flow, coronary vasomotion, and vasodilator capacity. Circulation 1998; 98: 119–25.
34. Heller LI, Cates C, Popma J et al. Intracoronary Doppler assessment of moderate coronary artery disease: comparison with 201Tl imaging and coronary angiography. Circulation 1997; 96: 484–90.
35. Vogel RA. Assessing stenosis significance by coronary arteriography. Are the best variables good enough? J Am Coll Cardiol 1988; 12: 692–3.

36. Serruys PW, Di Mario C, Piek J et al. Prognostic value of intracoronary flow velocity and diameter stenosis in assessing the short- and long-term outcomes of coronary balloon angioplasty: the Debate Study (Doppler Endpoints Balloon Angioplasty Trial Europe). Circulation 1997; 96: 3369–77.

37. Scheuble A, Feldman LJ, Brochet E et al. Measurement of coronary flow reserve by high-frequency transthoracic Doppler ultrasonography: indications and results. Arch Mal Coeur Vaiss 2003; 96(5): 25–33.

38. Saraste M, Koshenvuo JW, Mikkola J et al. Technical achievement: transthoracic Doppler echocardiography can be used to detect LAD restenosis after coronary angioplasty. Clin Physiol 2000; 20: 428–33.

39. Matsumura Y, Hozumi T, Watanabe H et al. Cut-off value of coronary flow velocity reserve by transthoracic Doppler echocardiography for diagnosis of significant left anterior descending artery stenosis in patients with coronary risk factors. Am J Cardiol 2003; 92: 1389–93.

40. Ferrari M, Schnell B, Werner GS, Figulla HR. Safety of deferring angioplasty in patients with normal coronary flow velocity reserve. J Am Coll Cardiol 1999; 33: 82–7.

41. Okayama H, Sumimoto T, Hiasa G et al. Assessment of intermediate stenosis in the left anterior descending coronary artery with contrast-enhanced transthoracic color-Doppler echocardiography. Coron Artery Dis 2003; 14: 247–54.

42. Voci P, Pizzuto F, Mariano E et al. Measurement of coronary flow reserve in the anterior and posterior descending coronary arteries by transthoracic Doppler ultrasound. Am J Cardiol 2002; 90: 988–91.

43. Voci P, Pizzuto F, Mariano E et al. Usefulness of coronary flow reserve measured by transthoracic coronary Doppler ultrasound to detect severe left anterior descending coronary artery stenosis. Am J Cardiol 2003; 92: 1320–4.

44. Conrad WA. Pressure–flow relationship in collapsible tubes. IEEE 1969; 16: 284–95.

45. Seiler C, Fleisch M, Meier B. Direct intracoronary evidence of collateral steal in humans. Circulation 1997; 96: 4261–7.

46. Higashiue S, Watanabe H, Yokoi Y et al. Simple detection of severe coronary stenosis using transthoracic Doppler echocardiography at rest. Am J Cardiol 2001; 87: 1064–8.

47. Watanabe N, Akasaka T, Yamaura Y et al. Noninvasive detection of total occlusion of the left anterior descending coronary artery with transthoracic Doppler echocardiography. J Am Coll Cardiol 2001; 38: 1328–32.

48. Pizzuto F, Voci P, Puddu PE, Chiricolo G, Borzi M, Romeo F. Functional assessment of the collateral-dependent circulation in chronic total coronary occlusion using transthoracic Doppler ultrasound and venous adenosine infusion. Am J Cardiol 2006, 98: 197–203.

49. Rentrop KP, Cohen M, Blanke H et al. Changes in collateral channel filling immediately after controlled coronary artery occlusion by an angioplasty balloon in human subjects. J Am Coll Cardiol 1985; 5: 587–92.

50. Ilia R, Carmel S, Cafri C et al. Coronary collaterals in patients with normal and impaired left ventricular systolic function. Int J Cardiol 1998; 63: 151–3.

51. Ruscazio M, Montisci R, Colonna P et al. Detection of coronary restenosis after coronary angioplasty by contrast-enhanced transthoracic echocardiographic Doppler assessment of coronary flow velocity reserve. J Am Coll Cardiol 2002; 40: 896–903.

52. Pizzuto F, Voci P, Mariano E et al. Noninvasive coronary flow reserve assessed by trans-thoracic coronary Doppler ultrasound in patients with left anterior descending coronary artery stents. Am J Cardiol 2003; 91: 522–6.

53. Hozumi T, Yoshida K, Akasaka T et al. Value of acceleration flow and the prestenotic to stenotic coronary flow velocity ratio by transthoracic color Doppler echocardiography in noninvasive diagnosis of restenosis after percutaneous transluminal coronary angioplasty. J Am Coll Cardiol 2000; 35: 164–8.

54. Voci P, Pizzuto F. Coronary flow. How far can we go with echocardiography? J Am Coll Cardiol 2001; 38: 1885–7.

55. Crowley JJ, Shapiro LM. Noninvasive assessment of left internal mammary artery graft patency using transthoracic echocardiography. Circulation 1995; 92: II25–30.

56. Pezzano A, Fusco R, Child M et al. Assessment of left internal mammary artery grafts using dipyridamole Doppler echocardiography. Am J Cardiol 1997; 80: 1603–6.
57. Calafiore A, Gallina S, Iacò A et al. Minimally invasive mammary artery Doppler flow velocity evaluation in minimally invasive coronary operations. Ann Thorac Surg 1998; 66: 1236–41.
58. Pizzuto F, Voci P, Sinatra R et al. Non-invasive assessment of coronary flow velocity reserve before and after angioplasty in a patient with mammary graft stenosis. Ital Heart J 2000; 1: 636–9.
59. Pizzuto F, Voci P, Mariano E, Puddu PE, Aprile A, Romeo F. Evaluation of flow in the left anterior descending coronary artery but not in the left internal mammary artery graft predicts significant stenosis of the arterial conduit. J Am Coll Cardiol 2005; 45: 424–32.
60. Roberts WC, Gardin JM. Location of myocardial infarcts: a confusion of terms and definitions. Am J Cardiol 1978; 868–72.
61. Udelson JE, Heller GV, Wackers FJ et al. Randomized, controlled dose-ranging study of the selective adenosine A_{2A} receptor agonist binodenoson for pharmacological stress as an adjunct to myocardial perfusion imaging. Circulation 2004; 109: 457–64.
62. Voci P, Mariano E, Pizzuto F et al. Coronary recanalization in anterior myocardial infarction. The open perforator hypothesis. J Am Coll Cardiol 2002; 40: 1205–13.
63. Lepper W, Hoffmann R, Kamp O et al. Assessment of myocardial reperfusion by intravenous myocardial contrast echocardiography and coronary flow reserve after primary percutaneous transluminal coronary angiography in patients with acute myocardial infarction. Circulation 2000; 101: 2368–74.
64. Yamamoto K, Ito H, Iwakura K et al. Two different coronary blood flow velocity patterns in thrombolysis in myocardial infarction flow grade 2 in acute myocardial infarction. Insight into mechanisms of microvascular dysfunction. J Am Coll Cardiol 2002; 40: 1755–60.
65. Yamamuro A, Akasaka T, Tamita K et al. Coronary flow velocity pattern immediately after percutaneous coronary intervention as a predictor of complications and in-hospital survival after acute myocardial infarction. Circulation 2002; 106: 3051–6.
66. Kajiya F, Matsuoka S, Ogasawara Y et al. Velocity profiles and phasic flow patterns in the non-stenotic human left anterior descending coronary artery during cardiac surgery. Cardiovasc Res 1993; 27: 845–50.
67. Di Mario C, Krams R, Serruys PV et al. Slope of instantaneous hyperemic diastolic coronary flow velocity–pressure relation. A new index for assessment of the physiological significance of coronary stenosis in humans. Circulation 1994; 90: 1215–24.
68. Tachibana K, Tachibana S. Albumin microbubble echo-contrast material as an enhancer of ultrasound accelerated thrombolysis. Circulation 1995; 92: 1148–50.
69. Unger EC, Matsunaga TO, McCreery T, et al. Therapeutic applications of microbubbles. Eur J Radiol 2002; 42: 160–8.
70. Distante A, Dankowski R, Mincarone P et al. Contrast echocardiography and medical economics: looking into the crystall ball. Eur Heart J 2002; 4(Suppl C): C39–47.
71. Malekianpour M, Rodés J, Coté G et al. Value of exercise electrocardiography in the detection of restenosis after coronary angioplasty in patients with one-vessel disease. Am J Cardiol 1999; 84: 258–63.
72. Beygui F, Le Feuvre C, Maunoury C et al. Detection of coronary restenosis by exercise electrocardiography thallium-201 perfusion imaging and coronary angiography in asymptomatic patients after percutaneous transluminal coronary angioplasty. Am J Cardiol 2000; 86: 35–40.
73. Heinle SK, Lieberman EB, Ancukiewiz M et al. Usefulness of dobutamine echocardiography for detecting restenosis after percutaneous transluminal coronary angioplasty. Am J Cardiol 1993; 72: 1220–5.
74. Riou LM, Ruiz M, Rieger JM et al. Influence of propranolol, enalaprilat, verapamil, and caffeine on adenosine A_{2A} receptor-mediated coronary vasodilation. J Am Coll Cardiol 2002; 40: 1687–94.
75. Pizzuto F, Voci P, Romeo F. Value of echocardiography in predicting future cardiac events after acute myocardial infarction. Curr Opin Cardiol 2003; 18: 378–84.

76. Rigo F, Cortigiani L, Pasanisi E et al. The additional prognostic value of coronary flow reserve on left anterior descending artery in patients with negative stress echo by wall motion criteria. A transthoracic vasodilator stress echocardiography study. Am Heart J 2006; 151: 124–30.
77. Voci P, Testa G, Plaustro G, Caretta Q. Coronary Doppler intensity changes during hand-grip: a new method to detect coronary vasomotor tone in coronary artery disease. J Am Coll Cardiol 1999; 34: 428–34.
78. Feinstein SB, Voci P, Pizzuto F. Noninvasive surrogate markers of atherosclerosis. Am J Cardiol 2002; 89: 31C–44C.

4

Non-invasive coronary angiography using multidetector computed tomography

Francesco Pizzuto and Paolo Voci

Use of MDCT for coronary angiography • Screening for coronary artery disease
• Follow-up of coronary therapeutic interventions • Coronary artery anomalies
• Non-calcified plaque • Hybrid nuclear/CT imaging • Radiation exposure
• Conclusion

Coronary angiography using contrast-enhanced multidetector computed tomography (MDCT) is a non-invasive technique that allows, for the first time, imaging of both the lumen and the wall of the coronary arteries from their origin at the aortic root to their very distal tract. The technique is currently used for the detection of obstructive coronary artery disease in patients with multiple risk factors and/or with symptoms, and to control the results of percutaneous coronary intervention or bypass surgery.

MDCT has several advantages with respect to electronic beam computed tomography (EBCT), which is mainly used for calcium score assessment as a surrogate marker of coronary atherosclerosis. Compared to EBCT, MDCT has a higher power, which becomes important in larger patients, and thinner slice imaging, with a section thickness as small as 0.5 mm whereas EBCT is limited to 1.5 mm. Conversely, EBCT delivers lower radiation doses compared to MDCT angiography (1.1 to 1.5 mSv vs 5 to 13 mSv, respectively).[1,2] The increase in resolution of CT is obtained at the expense of a higher radiation exposure, but the radiation dose estimates are likely to decrease with modification of the hardware design and scanning protocols. The clinical relevance of the radiation dose that is administered with cardiac CT is unclear. However, higher radiation doses in general are associated with a small but definite increase in cancer risk later in life.

An area of ongoing clinical research is the application of hybrid CT scanners integrating either positron emission tomography CT (PET-CT) or single photon emission computed tomography (SPECT-CT). These applications will allow for the acquisition of metabolic and perfusion information simultaneously with anatomic data on coronary artery morphology and coronary calcium. However, the incremental benefit of these new hybrid imaging strategies needs to be demonstrated before a widespread clinical use may be recommended, as radiation exposure may be significantly increased with the association of nuclear and CT imaging.

USE OF MDCT FOR CORONARY ANGIOGRAPHY

Initial studies with 4-detector systems demonstrated the ability of mechanical CT scanners to visualize the coronary arteries.[3-12] However, spatial and temporal resolution were severely limited and resulting artifacts, mainly due to coronary wall calcifications, precluded image evaluation regarding the presence of hemodynamically significant stenoses in up to 30% of cases. The introduction of 16-detector systems, which combined submillimeter collimation with faster gantry rotation times, definitely improved image definition. Consequently, the accuracy of CT angiography for detecting and ruling out hemodynamically relevant coronary artery stenoses increased substantially, with sensitivities ranging from 72 to 98% and specificities from 86 to 98%.[13-28]

The current use of 64-detector MDCT, by the increased collimation width and greater number of slices obtained, allows for shorter examination times by reducing both the breathhold time and the volume of contrast agent required. However, the acquisition speed is not much faster than that of 16-detector scanners, with the fastest gantry rotation currently at 330 ms. Several single-center studies of 64-row MDCT for the detection of coronary artery stenoses have reported excellent results, with overall reported sensitivities ranging between 95 and 99% and specificities between 93 and 96%.[29-34] Subset analysis, however, confirms that patients with Agastone calcium scores above 400, obesity, and a heart rate above 70 beats/min remain a diagnostic problem. For all MDCT scanner generations, including 64-row CT, it has been repeatedly shown that low heart rates significantly improve image quality and evaluability.[35-38] Another advantage of low heart rate is that it allows better application of algorithms that modulate the X-ray tube current in synchronization with the patient's ECG to reduce unnecessary radiation exposure in systole.[39,40] Therefore, a low heart rate (preferably below 60 beats/min) is desirable for MDCT imaging of the coronary arteries, and pretreatment with beta-blockers is often used for this purpose. Because of the need for retrospective gating for MDCT angiography, atrial fibrillation and other irregular heart rhythms remain a contraindication. In addition, the occasional occurrence of an ectopic beat during image acquisition may produce artifacts affecting complete reading of the test (Figure 4.1).

A meta-analysis[41] confirmed the clinical evidence that MDCT has a higher diagnostic accuracy when compared with magnetic resonance angiography. Another recent meta-analysis[42] reported the diagnostic accuracy of MDCT by a patient and coronary segments analysis. According to this study, average sensitivity is higher for proximal stenosis (90%, Figure 4.2) when compared to distal segments (80%), whereas specificity values are similar (90%) for proximal, mid, and distal segments.[42]

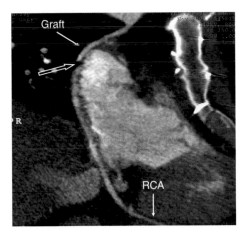

Figure 4.1 Patient with autologous saphenous vein grafted to the right coronary artery (RCA). An artifact (empty arrow) due to a premature ventricular beat does not allow adequate visualization of the graft, preventing any clinical conclusion.

SCREENING FOR CORONARY ARTERY DISEASE

Several studies defined the accuracy of MDCT coronary angiography for the assessment of coronary artery stenoses and convincingly demonstrated a very high negative predictive value of CT coronary angiography. Therefore, a 'normal' CT coronary angiogram permits exclusion of the presence of a significant coronary artery stenosis with a high degree of certainty (Figure 4.3). In the clinical arena, this high negative predictive value may be useful to avoid

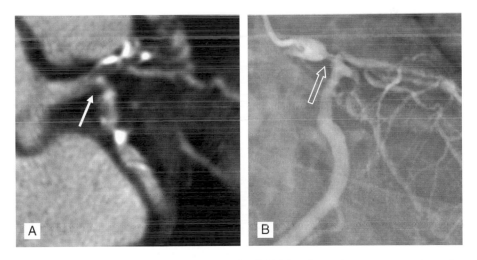

Figure 4.2 Multidetector computed tomography (MDCT) and invasive coronary angiography of a patient with effort chest pain and left ventricle bundle block (LVBB). The LVBB prevented the use of stress tests. The MDCT (A) showed a significant stenosis of the distal left main trunk (white arrow), which was confirmed by invasive angiography (B, open arrow).

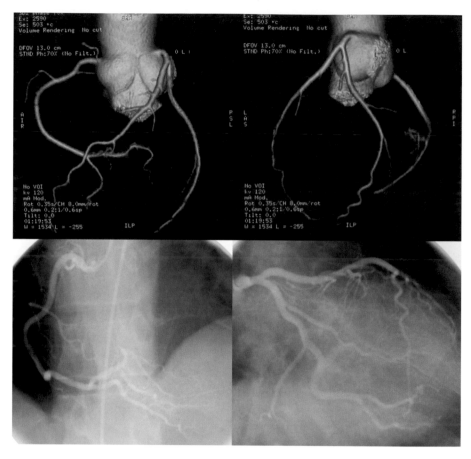

Figure 4.3   Upper panels: 64-slice multidetector computed tomography of a patient with chest pain shows absence of coronary atherosclerosis. Lower panels: invasive coronary angiography confirms the absence of coronary luminal narrowing.

invasive coronary angiography in patients whose symptoms or abnormal stress tests make it necessary to rule out coronary artery stenoses (Figure 4.4).[43] CT coronary angiography appears to be reasonable also for the assessment of obstructive coronary artery disease in symptomatic patients (Figures 4.5 to 4.9), even though the published series are limited to selected, stable patients with known or suspected coronary artery disease who were undergoing elective catheterization.[13–34] In these studies, results are generally limited to relatively large vessel sizes (≥1.5 mm), but the inclusion of smaller or uninterpretable vessels may reduce the sensitivity. However, CT angiography has a low accuracy for quantitating the degree of a coronary luminal narrowing, a surrogate index of physiologic impact. Recent studies with 64-slice CT indicate that quantitative estimates of stenosis severity by CT angiography correlate only modestly with quantitative coronary angiography (Figure 4.10).[24,30,31] This difference can be explained by the limited spatial and temporal resolution of MDCT, compared

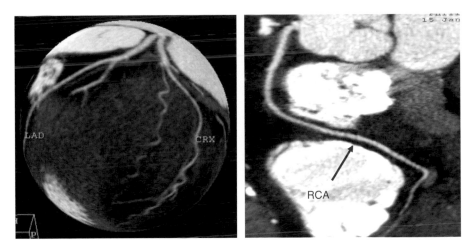

Figure 4.4 Patient with typical chest pain and normal computed tomography coronary angiography. The information was sufficient to rule out the presence of significant obstructive coronary artery disease and the need for invasive coronary angiography. LAD, left anterior descending coronary artery; LCX, left circumflex coronary artery; RCA, right coronary artery.

with conventional coronary angiography, which leads to image degradation by motion and calcium. The bright, blooming signal from high-density objects such as calcific plaques magnifies their true size, thereby leading to overestimation of stenosis severity.[17,19] Although improvements in spatial resolution may decrease the blooming effect of calcified lesions, this would increase radiation dose. It is

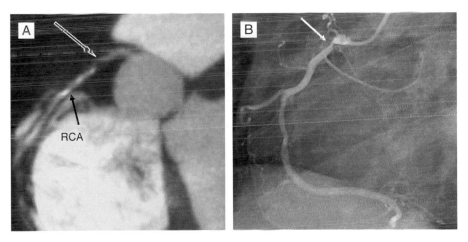

Figure 4.5 Patient with isolated episode of typical chest pain at rest, lasting 30 minutes, who arrived at the chest pain unit with normal EKG and without elevation of the cardiac enzymes. (A) Multidetector computed tomography shows the presence of a non-calcified critical obstructive lesion (open arrow) in the proximal segment of the right coronary artery (RCA). (B) Invasive coronary angiography confirms the findings of computed tomography (arrow).

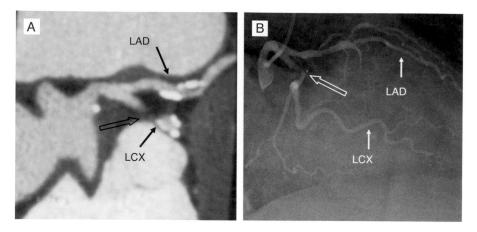

Figure 4.6   Patient with effort angina. (A) Multidetector computed tomography shows a calcified non-obstructive lesion in the proximal tract of the LAD and a mixed (fibrolipid and calcified) obstructive lesion (open black arrow) in the proximal LCX. (B) Invasive coronary angiography confirms the non significant luminal narrowing in the proximal LAD and a severe luminal obstruction in the LCX (open white arrow).

therefore clear that MDCT is superior for excluding obstructive coronary artery disease rather than predicting obstructive disease needing coronary revascularization.

The use of CT angiography in asymptomatic subjects as a screening test for atherosclerosis (Figure 4.11) is under investigation. Even tough preliminary

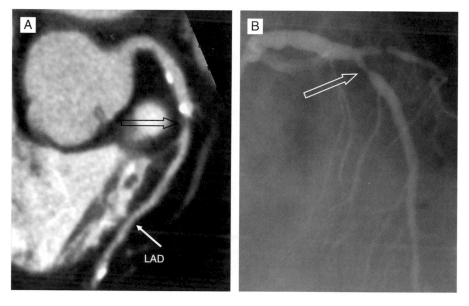

Figure 4.7   Patient with acute coronary syndrome. (A) Multidetector computed tomography shows a mixed (fibrolipid and calcified) obstructive lesion (open black arrow) in the proximal tract of the LAD. (B) Invasive coronary angiography confirms the significant luminal narrowing of the LAD (open white arrow).

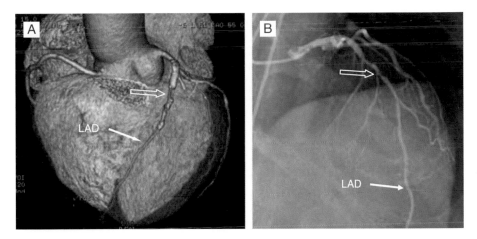

Figure 4.8 Patient with isolated episode of typical chest pain at rest, lasting 15 minutes. (A) Multidetector computed tomography (volume rendering mode) shows the presence of a mixed (calcified and fibrolipid) significant lesion in the middle segment (open arrow) of the LAD. (B) Invasive coronary angiography confirms the findings of computed tomography.

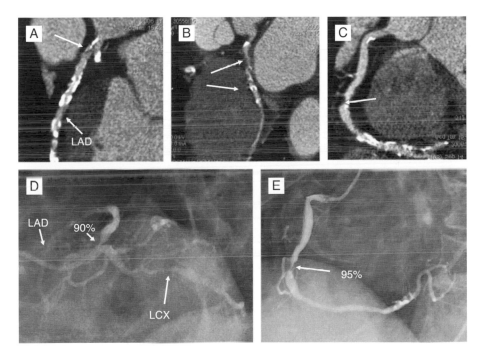

Figure 4.9 Patient with a history of hypertension and recent episodes of effort angina. Upper panels: multidetector computed tomography. (A) A critical mixed (fibrolipid and calcified) lesion (arrow) is visualized at the take-off of the LAD. A large amount of calcium is present in the LAD after the lesion. (B) The LCX also shows a significant mixed lesion in its proximal tract (arrows). (C) The RCA shows a subocclusive, fibrolipid plaque at the level of the middle segment (arrow), followed by a long, non-obstructive calcium deposition in the distal segment. Lower panels: invasive coronary angiography. The lesions of the LAD and the LCX are confirmed (F), as well as the subocclusion of the RCA (F).

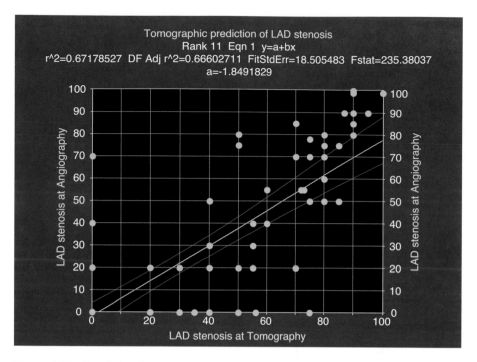

Figure 4.10 Correlation between quantitative coronary angiography (QCA) and 64-slice computed tomography angiography measurements of diameter stenosis in diseased coronary artery segments. Pearson's correlation coefficient $r=0.54$. Reproduced with permission from Leber et al.[31]

results are encouraging,[44] age may be a limiting factor for the high probability of encountering coronary calcifications. To date, the use of CT angiography as a screening test for atherosclerosis in asymptomatic subjects has not been recommended (Class III, Level of Evidence: C) by a recent ad hoc committee of the American Heart Association.[45] However, the evidence supporting the role of assessment of ischemia versus anatomy must be considered. Data from the Coronary Artery Surgery Study (CASS) registry have shown that, even in the setting of anatomic multivessel coronary artery disease, a survival benefit from revascularization compared with medical therapy only occurred in the setting of ECG evidence of ischemia, poor exercise tolerance, or both.[46,47]

Finally, 64-slice cardiac CT angiography has been suggested for diagnosing acute coronary syndromes and predicting clinical outcome in patients reaching the emergency department with a chest pain of uncertain origin.[48] In this series, MDCT sensitivity for predicting major adverse cardiac events (death, myocardial infarction, or revascularization) during hospitalization and follow-up was 92%, specificity was 76%, positive predictive value was 52%, and negative predictive value was 97%.[48]

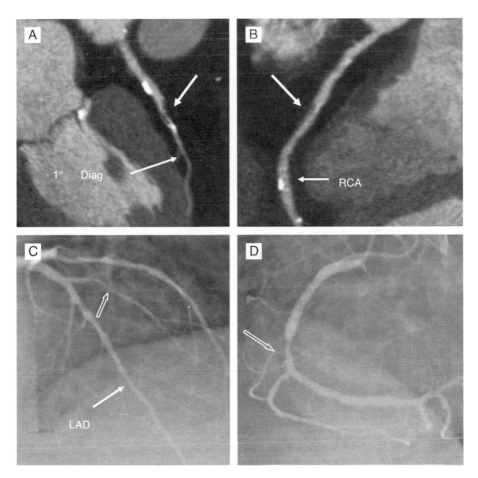

Figure 4.11   Asymptomatic patient with dyslipidemia and previous percutaneous intervention in the left Iliac artery. Upper panels: multidetector computed tomography. A mixed, fibrolipid and calcific, plaque (arrow) at the level of the first diagonal branch (A) and a fibrolipid (soft) plaque (arrow) in the middle tract of the RCA (B) are shown. Lower panels: invasive coronary angiography. A significant luminal narrowing (open arrow) of the first diagonal branch (C) and a significant luminal narrowing (open arrow) of the RCA, middle tract (D), are confirmed. LAD, left anterior descending coronary artery; RCA, right coronary artery; DIAG, diagonal branch.

FOLLOW-UP OF CORONARY THERAPEUTIC INTERVENTIONS

Percutaneous coronary intervention

Several studies, but of small sample size, have assessed the ability of MDCT in the detection of restenosis after coronary stenting. However, the use of 4- and 16-detector MDCT was of limited value as artifacts, caused by stent materials, often prevented adequate visualization of the coronary lumen within the stent.[49-54] Image quality for visualizing in-stent restenosis depends on stent characteristics, namely its design, material and size, and scanner technology (Figures 4.12-4.14).[55-57] In one recent study performed by 64-slice CT the sensitivity for

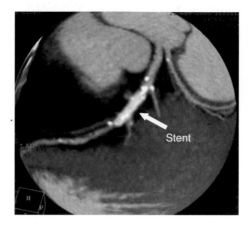

Figure 4.12   Patient with an old bare metal stent implant in the middle tract of the LAD. The blooming of the stented segment during multislice computed tomography does not allow the correct evaluation of the patency of the stent.

detection of in-stent restenosis was 83%, despite this only 8 stenoses were found, thus preventing a reliable clinical application of the method in patients with coronary stents.

Bypass artery surgery

Numerous studies have shown that MDCT allows reliable imaging of coronary artery bypass graft patency and occlusion, with the accuracy to detect bypass occlusion approaching 100%.[55-75] Alone, this information about patency is not sufficient; we also need to know whether there are lesions along the graft, the

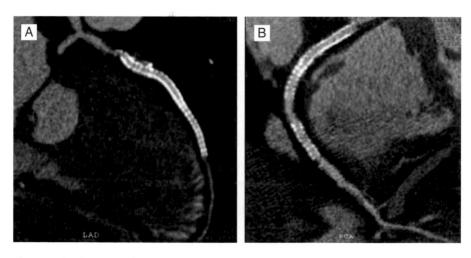

Figure 4.13   Patient with multiple bare metal stents, recently implanted at the level of the middle and distal tracts of the LAD (A) and of the middle and distal tracts of the RCA (B). The stent structure allows an adequate analysis of the internal lumen of the stented segments, which appear patent and without intraluminal neointimal hyperplasia.

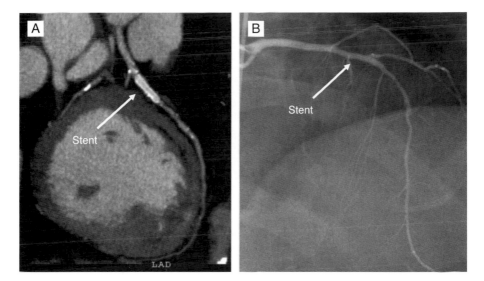

Figure 4.14 Patient with a recent stenting of the middle segment of the LAD. Multidetector computed tomography (A) allows a careful evaluation of the stent, without in-stent hyperplasia and/or restenosis. The invasive coronary angiogram (B) confirms the computed tomography findings.

suture site and the native coronary vessel (Figures 4.15-4.19). The graft is larger and is less affected by translational and rotational movements of the beating heart, than a native coronary artery. It is therefore not surprising that the graft is better imaged than the native vessel. Nevertheless, artifacts caused by metal clips may also shadow segments of the graft. This is more difficult, owing to the smaller caliber of these vessels (Figure 4 20), hence, more data is necessary, and newer scanners may have the spatial resolution to overcome some of the earlier problems with graft and native coronary vessel assessment.

CORONARY ARTERY ANOMALIES

Anomalous coronary arteries can be found in patients with suspected coronary disease, chest pain, syncope, or sudden death. The visualization of the origin and the course of anomalous coronary arteries may be difficult with invasive coronary angiography, due to its two-dimensional nature. Conversely, MDCT allows a three-dimensional imaging of the coronary arteries, with easy detection of the origin and course of anomalous vessels.[76-81] Compared to magnetic resonance imaging, which also allows visualization of coronary anomalies, CT requires radiation and a contrast agent. However, MDCT is superior in terms of spatial and temporal resolution and the speed of image acquisition.

NON-CALCIFIED PLAQUE

A unique feature of MDCT as a non-invasive tool is the potential for visualization and characterization of coronary artery plaques. Soft plaques may be at increased risk for erosion or rupture even when they do not produce a significant degree of luminal stenosis, and they are thought to play a role in the

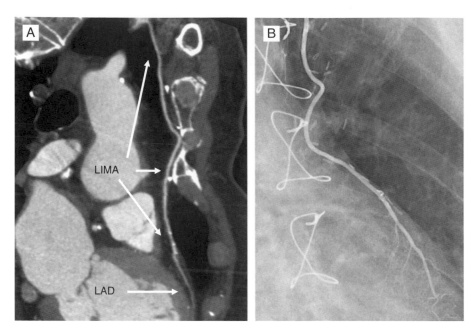

Figure 4.15   Patient with well-functioning left internal mammary artery (LIMA) grafted to the LAD. Multidetector computed tomography (A) clearly shows a patent LIMA grafted to the middle tract of the LAD. The anastomotic site is well preserved, and the post-anastomotic distal LAD is fully patent. Invasive coronary angiography (B) confirms the non-invasive findings.

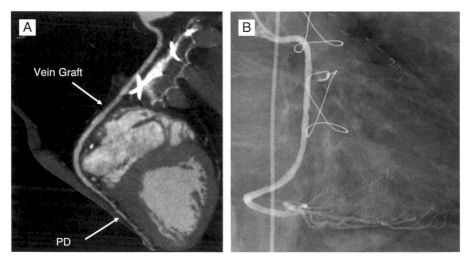

Figure 4.16   Well-functioning vein graft from aortic root to the RCA, clearly documented by multidetector computed tomography (A), and confirmed by invasive coronary angiography (B). PD, posterior descending coronary artery.

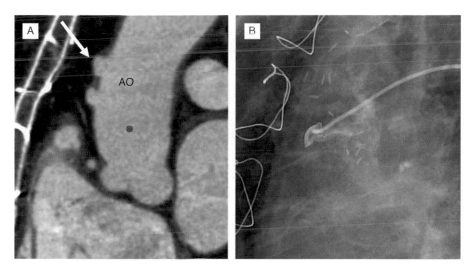

Figure 4.17   Patient with proximally occluded coronary vein graft from aorta to obtuse marginal branch. Multidetector computed tomography (A) showed an occluded vein graft (arrow), originating from the anterior wall of the ascending aorta (AO). Invasive coronary angiography (B) confirmed the remnant of a vein graft.

development of acute coronary ischemic events (Figures 4.5 and 4.7). Coronary angiography is the standard imaging modality to evaluate coronary artery disease. However, both autopsy and coronary intravascular ultrasound imaging studies have shown that angiographically 'normal' coronary artery segments may contain a significant amount of atherosclerotic plaque. In these cases

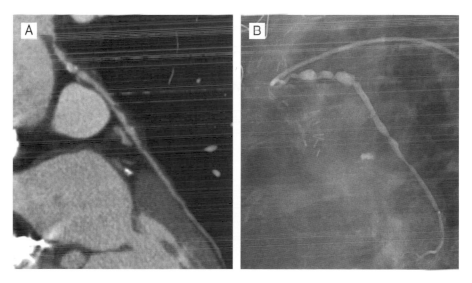

Figure 4.18   Patient with multiple stenoses in the proximal and middle segments of a vein graft from aorta to the first obtuse marginal branch of the LCX, shown by multidetector computed tomography (A) and confirmed by invasive coronary angiography (B).

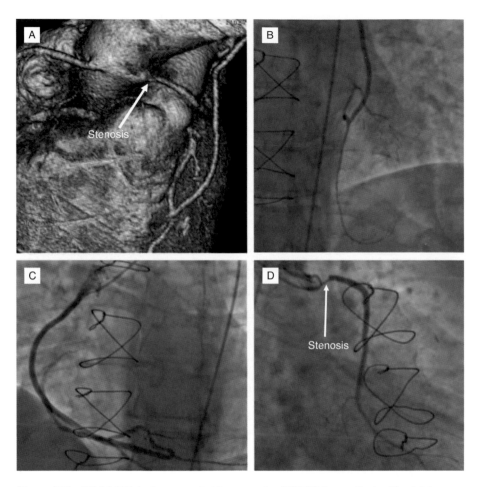

Figure 4.19   (A) Multidetector computed tomography (MDCT) in a patient with a triple coronary artery bypass graft. A comprehensive view shows all grafts: a well functioning left internal mammary artery grafted to the LAD, a well-functioning autologous saphenous vein grafted to the RCA, and an autologous saphenous vein grafted to the first obtuse marginal branch, with a ignificant proximal stenosis (arrow). Invasive selective coronary angiography (from B to D) confirms the MDCT findings.

coronary angiography, used to evaluate the internal coronary lumen, may underestimate the extent of coronary atherosclerosis, due to positive remodelling of the coronary vessel.[82-83] Improved spatial and temporal image acquisition with submillimeter slice collimation has facilitated atherosclerotic plaque detection with MDCT. The so-called unstable plaques generally have a high lipid content, and can be detected as low-density lesions on MDCT, whereas structures with densities above the adjacent vessel lumen are considered calcified (Figure 4.21).[86] Three types of plaque have been identified:

(1) 'soft' plaque, presumably lipid laden with lower densities
(2) intermediate or presumably fibrous plaques and
(3) calcific or high-density plaques.

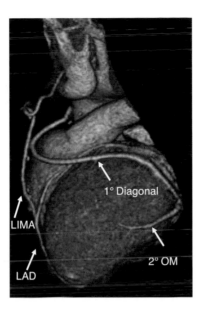

Figure 4.20 3D volume rendering of a patient with a LIMA grafted to the LAD, and a sequential vein grafted from the aorta to the 1° diagonal branch of the LAD and the 2° obtuse marginal branch (OM) of the LCX. The LIMA–LAD graft, its joining tract with the LAD, as well as the postanastomotic LAD tract appear well functioning. The sequential vein graft is fully open and the OM is well visualized, without any stenosis. The 1° diagonal branch after the anastomosis with the vein graft is scarcely seen because of its small caliber, and it cannot adequately be described.

MDCT allows accurate detection and differentiation of coronary plaque when compared with intravascular ultrasound, which is currently the gold-standard technique for plaque characterization.[87–91] Sensitivities for detection of hypoechoic, lipid-rich non-calcified plaque by MDCT may range from 50 to 90%. As expected, the sensitivities for detecting calcific atheroma were higher (approximately 88 to 95%) than for non calcific plaques. These studies demonstrate the diagnostic potentiality of MDCT in characterizing noncalcific atheroma, with some uncertainty in discriminating lipid-laden and fibrous components. Quantification of coronary atherosclerotic plaque burden by CT technology is currently unsatisfactory,[92] as MDCT substantially underestimated plaque volume compared to intravascular ultrasound.[87,93] In addition, the reproducibility of the measure has not been reported. Finally, this procedure requires both contrast administration and radiation exposure, and the risks may overcome the benefit in individual patients.

HYBRID NUCLEAR/CT IMAGING

Functional information demonstrating the physiologic significance of coronary lesions is important for clinical decision-making related to revascularization. The presence of a large amount of calcium within the wall of the coronary artery may prevent the correct interpretation of MDCT by masking the presence of

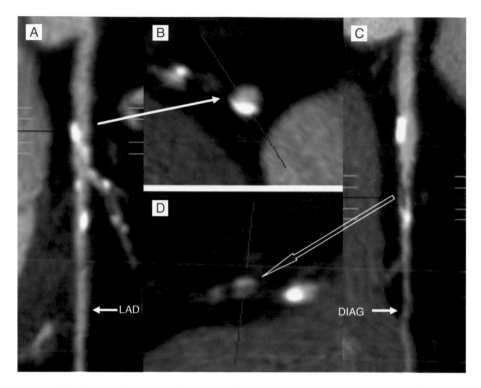

Figure 4.21   Plaque characterization by multidetector computed tomography. (A) The linear reconstruction of the LAD shows a non-obstructive calcified plaque at its middle tract. (B) The cross-sectional tomographic image, obtained at the same level, shows a partially preserved internal lumen (arrow). (C) The linear reconstruction of the first diagonal branch (DIAG) shows a mixed (calcified and fibrolipidic) plaque. (D) The cross-section obtained at the same level shows a low-density (high lipid content) lesion (arrow), obstructing the arterial lumen.

significant endoluminal plaque in many cases (Figures 4.22 to 4.24). In these cases, the problem may be overcome by coupling morphologic and functional information (hybrid PET-CT and SPECT-CT scanners) which allow for the acquisition of metabolic and/or perfusion information along with angiographic data. Hybrid imaging is still a research tool with ongoing problems with image acquisition. However, growing and consistent evidence suggests that anatomy-based predictions of physiologic significance by CT coronary angiography differ substantially from direct measures of inducible myocardial ischemia, as assessed by myocardial perfusion imaging.[94–97] In the future, hybrid imaging strategies will allow for a more accurate definition of anatomic and physiologic components in a single test.[98] In cases of non-interpretable scans and/or in the presence of a large amount of calcium, the combination of coronary anatomy detection (MDCT) with transthoracic coronary Doppler echocardiography, enabling measurement of the physiologic impact of the stenosis by coronary flow velocity reserve, may be useful (Figures 4.25 and 4.26).

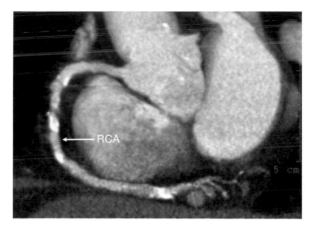

Figure 4.22 Patient with atypical angina. The large amount of calcium in the middle tract of the RCA and before its distal bifurcation prevents any information from being obtained on the internal lumen of the RCA.

RADIATION EXPOSURE

CT uses ionizing radiation to generate tomographic images. Although all individuals are exposed to ionizing radiation from natural sources every day, people involved in healthcare, particularly if dealing with medical imaging, must understand the potential risks of each test and balance them against the benefits. This is particularly important for tests given to healthy individuals as part of a disease-screening or a risk-stratification program.

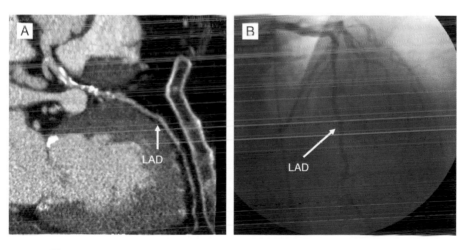

Figure 4.23 Patient with effort angina and an inconclusive effort EKG test. (A) Multidetector computed tomography (MDCT) showed a large amount of calcium within the proximal and middle tracts of the LAD, preventing adequate information from being obtained on the narrowing of the lumen of the artery. (B) Invasive coronary angiography showed the absence of the internal lumen narrowing of the LAD. The calcium seen with MDCT was entirely distributed within the external walls of the LAD.

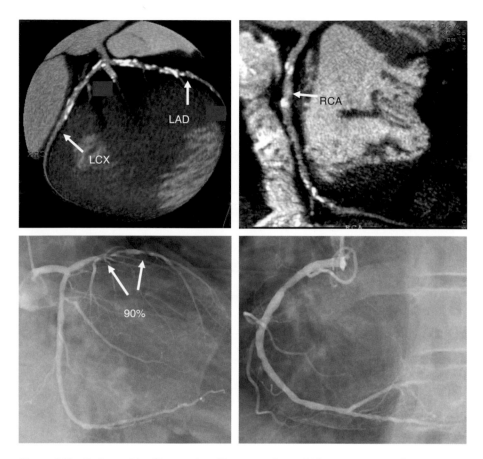

Figure 4.24   Patient with effort angina. Upper panels: multidetector computed tomography (MDCT). The 2D scans showed a large amont of calcium at the level of all the three main branches of the coronary arteries, preventing any information from being obtained about the internal lumen. Lower panels: invasive coronary angiography. The LAD had a tandem 90% stenosis of its proximal and middle tracts (arrows), which were undetectable with MDCT. The LCX and the RCA were free of significant lumen narrowing, a finding missed with MDCT.

In the field of radiation protection, the FDA states that the risk for adverse health effects from cancer is proportional to the amount of radiation dose absorbed, and the amount of dose depends on the type of X-ray examination.[99] A CT examination with an effective dose of 10 mSv may be associated with an increased chance of developing fatal cancer of approximately 1/2000. This may be a small number when compared with the natural prevalence of cancer in the general population, but it may turn out to be a public health concern if large numbers of the population undergo increased numbers of CT procedures for screening purposes.

The estimated dose from a chest X-ray is 0.04 to 0.10 mSv, and the average annual background radiation adsorbed by an individual in the United States is 3

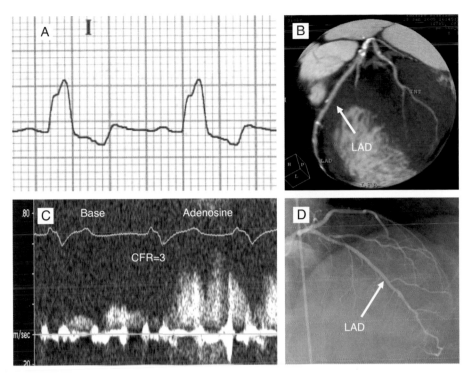

Figure 4.25 Patient with atypical chest pain. (A) An EKG left bundle block was present, which prevents the use of stress tests. (B) The multidetector computed tomography is inconclusive for the presence of a large amount of calcium at the proximal tract of the LAD. (C) A non-invasive coronary flow reserve (CFR) of 3, assessed by transthoracic coronary Doppler and venous adenosine infusion, excluded any significant narrowing along the LAD. (D) The invasive coronary angiography confirms the absence of any significant narrowing of the LAD.

to 3.6 mSv.[2] One drawback of MDCT is the high radiation exposure to the patient.[2,3,100-111] MDCT angiography requires retrospective gating, which is associated with significantly greater radiation exposures, to acquire images. Newer MDCT protocols allow for increased power utilization, with settings as high as 900 mA, which may deliver up to 11 to 13 mSv per study. Comparing different coronary imaging modalities, EBCT delivers 1.1 to 2.0 mSv, MDCT 8 to 18 mSv, and coronary angiography 2.1 to 2.3 mSv.[1,2,104-107] Interestingly, cardiac nuclear imaging has similar radiation exposure doses (8 to 12 mSv) to MDCT.[108] Specifically, technetium scintigraphy delivers the 'lowest' (6 to 8 mSv) and thallium the 'highest' (27 mSv) radiations.[109] With the retrospective ECG-gating mode scan data are acquired for the entire cardiac cycle, but in most cases the scan data used for image reconstruction are selected only in diastole. Therefore, a high tube current is required only in diastole. Tube current modulation with prospective ECG control (dose modulation) reduces radiation exposure substantially without decreasing image quality,[110,111] an effect that is more pronounced

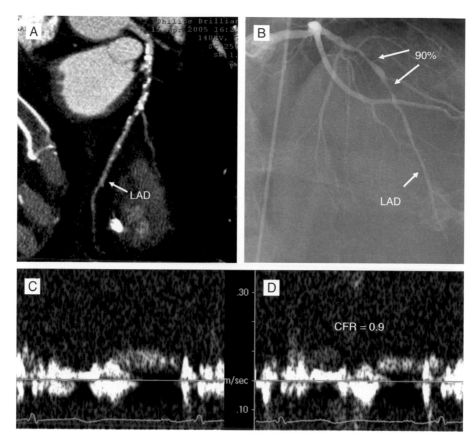

Figure 4.26   Patient with typical chest pain. (A) Multidetector computed tomography showed a large amount of calcium in the proximal and middle tracts of the LAD, which prevented any conclusion from being drawn on the internal lumen of the coronary artery. (B) Invasive coronary angiography documented the presence of a tandem 90% stenosis at the level of the proximal and middle tracts of the LAD. (C and D) Impaired non-invasive CFR of 0.9, obtained with transthoracic coronary Doppler ultrasound and venous adenosine infusion, predicted a subocclusion of the LAD. In this patient the combination of the two non-invasive tecnhiques was very useful to assess the significant LAD lesion.

for lower heart rates. Also, using the lowest necessary mA during each study will also help limit radiation exposure during these procedures.

CONCLUSION

CT technology has definitely entered as a useful new diagnostic tool in cardiology. The technology is evolving rapidly and radiation exposures are likely to be reduced with modification of the hardware and scanning protocols. For MDCT, increased numbers of detectors allow for better collimation and spatial reconstruction. Having more of the heart visualized simultaneously will also allow for reductions in the contrast requirements and breathholding for the patient, further improving the methodology.

REFERENCES

1. Morin RL, Gerber TC, McCollough CH. Radiation dose in computed tomography of the heart. Circulation 2003; 107: 917–22.
2. Hunold P, Vogt FM, Schmermund A et al. Radiation exposure during cardiac CT: effective doses at multi-detector row CT and electron-beam CT. Radiology 2003; 226: 145–52.
3. Achenbach S, Ulzheimer S, Baum U et al. Noninvasive coronary angiography by retrospectively ECG-gated multislice spiral CT. Circulation 2000; 102: 2823–8.
4. Nieman K, Oudkerk M, Rensing BJ et al. Coronary angiography with multi-slice computed tomography. Lancet 2001; 357: 599–603.
5. Achenbach S, Giesler T, Ropers D et al. Detection of coronary artery stenoses by contrast-enhanced, retrospectively electrocardiographically-gated, multi-slice spiral computed tomography. Circulation 2001; 103: 2535–8.
6. Knez A, Becker CR, Leber A et al. Usefulness of multislice spiral computed tomography angiography for determination of coronary artery stenoses. Am J Cardiol 2001; 88: 1191–4.
7. Vogl TJ, Abolmaali ND, Diebold T et al. Techniques for the detection of coronary atherosclerosis: multi-detector row CT coronary angiography. Radiology 2002; 223: 212–20.
8. Kopp AF, Schroeder S, Kuettner A et al. Non-invasive coronary angiography with high resolution multidetector-row computed tomography: results in 102 patients. Eur Heart J 2002; 23: 1714–25.
9. Nieman K, Rensing BJ, van Geuns RJ et al. Usefulness of multislice computed tomography for detecting obstructive coronary artery disease. Am J Cardiol 2002; 89: 913–8.
10. Becker CR, Knez A, Leber A et al. Detection of coronary artery stenoses with multislice helical CT angiography. J Comput Assist Tomogr 2002; 26: 750–5.
11. Morgan Hughes GJ, Marshall AJ, Roobottom CA. Multislice computed tomographic coronary angiography: experience in a UK centre. Clin Radiol 2003; 58: 378–83.
12. Sato Y, Matsumoto N, Kato M et al. Noninvasive assessment of coronary artery disease by multislice spiral computed tomography using a new retrospectively ECG-gated image reconstruction technique. Circ J 2003; 67: 401–5.
13. Maruyama T, Yoshizumi T, Tamura R et al. Comparison of visibility and diagnostic capability of noninvasive coronary angiography by eight slice multidetector-row computed tomography versus conventional coronary angiography. Am J Cardiol 2004; 93: 537–42.
14. Nieman K, Cademartiri F, Lemos PA et al. Reliable noninvasive coronary angiography with fast submillimeter multislice spiral computed tomography. Circulation 2002; 106: 2051–4.
15. Ropers D, Baum U, Pohle K et al. Detection of coronary artery stenoses with thin-slice multi detector row spiral computed tomography and multiplanar reconstruction. Circulation. 2003; 107: 664–6.
16. Kuettner A, Trabold T, Schroeder S et al. Noninvasive detection of coronary lesions using 16-detector multislice spiral computed tomography technology: initial clinical results. J Am Coll Cardiol 2004; 44: 1230–7.
17. Mollet NR, Cademartiri F, Nieman K et al. Multislice spiral computed tomography coronary angiography in patients with stable angina pectoris. J Am Coll Cardiol 2004; 43: 2265–70.
18. Martuscelli E, Romagnoli A, D'Eliseo A et al. Accuracy of thin-slice computed tomography in the detection of coronary stenoses. Eur Heart J 2004; 25: 1043–8.
19. Hoffmann U, Moselewski F, Cury RC et al. Predictive value of 16-slice multidetector spiral computed tomography to detect significant obstructive coronary artery disease in patients at high risk for coronary disease: patient versus segment-based analysis. Circulation 2004; 110: 2638–43.
20. Kuettner A, Beck T, Drosch T et al. Diagnostic accuracy of noninvasive coronary imaging using 16-detector slice spiral computed tomography with 188 ms temporal resolution. J Am Coll Cardiol 2005; 45: 123–7
21. Mollet NR, Cademartiri F, Krestin GP et al. Improved diagnostic accuracy with 16-row multi-slice computed tomography coronary angiography. J Am Coll Cardiol 2005; 45: 128–32.

22. Schuijf JD, Bax JJ, Salm LP et al. Noninvasive coronary imaging and assessment of left ventricular function using 16-slice computed tomography. Am J Cardiol 2005; 95: 571–4.
23. Morgan-Hughes GJ, Roobottom CA, Owens PE et al. Highly accurate coronary angiography with submillimetre, 16 slice computed tomography. Heart 2005; 91: 308–13.
24. Hoffmann MH, Shi H, Schmitz BL et al. Noninvasive coronary angiography with multislice computed tomography. JAMA 2005; 293: 2471–8.
25. Fine JJ, Hopkins CB, Hall PA, Delphia RE, Attebery TW, Newton FC. Noninvasive coronary angiography: agreement of multi-slice spiral computed tomography and selective catheter angiography. Int J Cardiovasc Imaging 2004; 20: 549–52.
26. Kaiser C, Bremerich J, Haller S et al. Limited diagnostic yield of non-invasive coronary angiography by 16-slice multidetector spiral computed tomography in routine patients referred for evaluation of coronary artery disease. Eur Heart J 2005; 26: 1987–92.
27. Aviram G, Finkelstein A, Herz I et al. Clinical value of 16-slice multi-detector CT compared to invasive coronary angiography. Int J Cardiovasc Intervent 2005; 7: 21–8.
28. Achenbach S, Ropers D, Pohle FK et al. Detection of coronary artery stenoses using multi-detector CT with 16 × 0.75 collimation and 375 ms rotation. Eur Heart J 2005; 26: 1978–86.
29. Leschka S, Alkadhi H, Plass A et al. Accuracy of MSCT coronary angiography with 64-slice technology: first experience. Eur Heart J 2005; 26: 1482–7.
30. Raff GL, Gallagher MJ, O'Neill WW et al. Diagnostic accuracy of noninvasive coronary angiography using 64-slice spiral computed tomography. J Am Coll Cardiol 2005; 46: 552–7.
31. Leber AW, Knez A, von Ziegler F et al. Quantification of obstructive and nonobstructive coronary lesions by 64-slice computed tomography: a comparative study with quantitative coronary angiography and intravascular ultrasound. J Am Coll Cardiol 2005; 46: 147–54.
32. Mollet NR, Cademartiri F, van Mieghem CA et al. High-resolution spiral computed tomography coronary angiography in patients referred for diagnostic conventional coronary angiography. Circulation 2005; 112: 2318–23.
33. Ropers D, Rixe J, Anders K et al. Usefulness of multidetector row computed tomography with 64-×0.6-mm collimation and 330-ms rotation for the noninvasive detection of significant coronary artery stenoses. Am J Cardiol 2006; 97: 343–8.
34. Fine JJ, Hopkins CB, Ruff N et al. Comparison of accuracy of 64-slice cardiovascular computed tomography with coronary angiography in patients with suspected coronary artery disease. Am J Cardiol 2006; 97: 173–4.
35. Giesler T, Baum U, Ropers D et al. Noninvasive visualization of coronary arteries using contrast-enhanced multidetector CT: influence of heart rate on image quality and stenosis detection. AJR 2002; 179: 911–6.
36. Schroeder S, Kopp AF, Kuettner A et al. Influence of heart rate on vessel visibility in non-invasive coronary angiography using new multislice computed tomography: experience in 94 patients. Clin Imaging 2002; 26: 106–11.
37. Hoffmann MH, Shi H, Manzke R et al. Noninvasive coronary angiography with 16-detector row CT: effect of heart rate. Radiology 2005; 234: 86–97.
38. Herzog C, Abolmaali N, Balzer JO et al. Heart-rate-adapted image reconstruction in multi-detector-row cardiac CT: influence of physiological and technical prerequisite on image quality. Eur Radiol 2002; 12: 2670–8.
39. Poll LW, Cohnen M, Brachten S et al. Dose reduction in multi-slice CT of the heart by use of ECG-controlled tube current modulation ('ECG pulsing'): phantom measurements. Eur Radiol 2002; 174: 1500–5.
40. Jakobs TF, Becker CR, Ohnesorge B et al. Multislice helical CT of the heart with retrospective ECG gating: reduction of radiation exposure by ECG-controlled tube current modulation. Eur Radiol 2002; 12: 1081–6.
41. Schuijf JD, Bax JJ, Shaw LJ et al. Meta-analysis of comparative diagnostic performance of magnetic resonance imaging and multislice computed tomography for noninvasive coronary angiography. Am Heart J 2006; 151: 404–11.
42. Stein PD, Beemath A, Kayali F et al. Multidetector computed tomography for the diagnosis of coronary artery disease: a systematic review. Am J Med 2006; 119: 203–16.

43. Gibbons RJ, Chatterjee K, Daley J et al. ACC/AHA/ACP-ASIM guidelines for the management of patients with chronic stable angina: executive summary and recommendations: a report of the American College of Cardiology/American Heart Association Task Force on Practice Guidelines (Committee on Management of Patients with Chronic Stable Angina). Circulation 1999; 99: 2829–48.

44. Romeo F, Leo R, Clementi F et al. Multislice computed tomography in an asymptomatic high-risk population. Am J Cardiol. 2007; 99: 325–8.

45. Budoff MJ, Achenbach S, Blumenthal RS et al. Assessment of coronary artery disease by cardiac computed tomography: a scientific statement from the American Heart Association Committee on Cardiovascular Imaging and Intervention, Council on Cardiovascular Radiology and Intervention, and Committee on Cardiac Imaging, Council on Clinical Cardiology. Circulation 2006; 114: 1761–91.

46. Weiner DA, Ryan TJ, McCabe CH et al. The role of exercise testing in identifying patients with improved survival after coronary artery bypass surgery. J Am Coll Cardiol 1986; 8: 741–8.

47. Wiener DA, Ryan TJ, McCabe CH et al. Value of exercise testing in determining the risk classification and the response to coronary artery bypass grafting in three-vessel coronary artery disease: a report from the Coronary Artery Surgery Study (CASS) registry. Am J Cardiol 1987; 60: 262–6

48. Rubinshtein R, Halon DA, Gaspar T et al. Usefulness of 64-slice cardiac computed tomographic angiography for diagnosing acute coronary syndromes and predicting clinical outcome in emergency department patients with chest pain of uncertain origin. Circulation 2007; 115: 1762–8

49. Pump H, Mohlenkamp S, Sehnert CA et al. Coronary arterial stent patency: assessment with electron-beam CT. Radiology 2000; 214: 447–52.

50. Gilard M, Cornily JC, Rioufol G et al. Noninvasive assessment of left main coronary stent patency with 16-slice computed tomography. Am J Cardiol 2005; 95: 110–12.

51. Hong C, Chrysant GS, Woodard PK et al. Coronary artery stent patency assessed with in-stent contrast enhancement measured at multi-detector row CT angiography: initial experience. Radiology 2004; 233: 286–91.

52. Knollmann FD, Moller J, Gebert A et al. Assessment of coronary artery stent patency by electron-beam CT. Eur Radiol 2004; 14: 1341–7.

53. Schuijf JD, Bax JJ, Jukema JW et al. Feasibility of assessment of coronary stent patency using 16-slice computed tomography. Am J Cardiol 2004; 94: 427–30.

54. Kruger S, Mahnken AH, Sinha AM et al. Multislice spiral computed tomography for the detection of coronary stent restenosis and patency. Int J Cardiol 89: 167–72.

55. Mahnken AH, Buecker A, Wildberger JE et al. Coronary artery stents in multislice computed tomography: in vitro artifact evaluation. Invest Radiol 2004; 39: 27–33.

56. Maintz D, Seifarth H, Flohr T et al. Improved coronary artery stent visualization and in-stent stenosis detection using 16-slice computed-tomography and dedicated image reconstruction technique. Invest Radiol 2003; 38: 790–5

57. Mahnken AH, Seyfarth T, Flohr T et al. Flat-panel detector computed tomography for the assessment of coronary artery stents: phantom study in comparison with 16-slice spiral computed tomography. Invest Radiol 2005; 40: 8–13.

58. Cademartiri F, Mollet N, Lemos PA et al. Usefulness of multislice computed tomographic coronary angiography to assess in-stent restenosis. Am J Cardiol 2005; 96: 799–802.

59. Stanford W, Brundage BH, MacMillan R et al. Sensitivity and specificity of assessing coronary bypass graft patency with ultrafast computed tomography: results of a multicenter study. J Am Coll Cardiol 1988; 12: 1–7.

60. Knez A, von Smekal A, Haberl R et al. The value of ultrafast computerized tomography in detection of the patency of coronary bypasses. Z Kardiol 1996; 85: 629–34.

61. Achenbach S, Moshage W, Ropers D et al. Noninvasive, three-dimensional visualization of coronary artery bypass grafts by electron beam tomography. Am J Cardiol 1997; 79: 856–61.

62. Ha JW, Cho SY, Shim WH et al. Noninvasive evaluation of coronary artery bypass graft patency using three-dimensional angiography obtained with contrast-enhanced electron beam CT. AJR 1999; 172: 1055–9.

63. Marano R, Storto ML, Maddestra N et al. Non-invasive assessment of coronary artery bypass graft with retrospectively ECG-gated four-row multi-detector spiral computed tomography. Eur Radiol 2004; 14: 1353–62.
64. Lu B, Dai RP, Zhuang N, Budoff MJ. Noninvasive assessment of coronary artery bypass graft patency and flow characteristics by electron-beam tomography. J Invasive Cardiol 2002; 14: 19–24.
65. Hoshi T, Yamauchi T, Kanauchi T et al. Three-dimensional computed tomography angiography of coronary artery bypass graft with electron beam tomography [in Japanese]. J Cardiol 2001; 38: 197–202.
66. Engelmann MG, von Smekal A, Knez A et al. Accuracy of spiral computed tomography for identifying arterial and venous coronary graft patency. Am J Cardiol 1997; 80: 569–74.
67. Burgstahler C, Kuettner A, Kopp AF et al. Non-invasive evaluation of coronary artery bypass grafts using multi-slice computed tomography: initial clinical experience. Int J Cardiol 2003; 90: 275–80.
68. Rossi R, Chiurlia E, Ratti C et al. Noninvasive assessment of coronary artery bypass graft patency by multislice computed tomography. Ital Heart J 2004; 5: 36–41.
69. Gurevitch J, Gaspar T, Orlov B et al. Noninvasive evaluation of arterial grafts with newly released multidetector computed tomography. Ann Thorac Surg 2003; 76: 1523–7.
70. Ropers D, Ulzheimer S, Wenkel E et al. Investigation of aortocoronary bypass grafts by multi-slice spiral computed tomography with electrocardiographic-gated image reconstruction. Am J Cardiol 2001; 88: 792–5.
71. Nieman K, Pattynama PM, Rensing BJ et al. Evaluation of patients after coronary artery bypass surgery: CT angiographic assessment of grafts and coronary arteries. Radiology 2003; 229: 749–56.
72. Martuscelli E, Romagnoli A, D'Eliseo A et al. Evaluation of venous and arterial conduit patency by 16-slice spiral computed tomography. Circulation 2004; 110: 3234–8.
73. Schlosser T, Konorza T, Hunold P et al. Noninvasive visualization of coronary artery bypass grafts using 16-detector row computed tomography. J Am Coll Cardiol 2004; 44: 1224–9.
74. Anders K, Baum U, Schmid M et al. Coronary artery bypass graft (CABG) patency: assessment with high-resolution submillimeter 16-slice multidetector-row computed tomography (MDCT) versus coronary angiography. Eur J Radiol 2006; 57: 336–44.
75. Chiurlia E, Menozzi M, Ratti C et al. Follow-up of coronary artery bypass graft patency by multislice computed tomography. Am J Cardiol 2005; 95: 1094–7.
76. Ropers D, Moshage W, Daniel WG et al. Visualization of coronary artery anomalies and their course by contrast-enhanced electron beam tomography and three-dimensional reconstruction. Am J Cardiol 2001; 87: 193–7.
77. Yoshimura N, Hamada S, Takamiya M et al. Coronary artery anomalies with a shunt: evaluation with electron-beam CT. J Comput Assist Tomogr. 1998; 22: 682–686.
78. Deibler AR, Kuzo RS, Vohringer M et al. Imaging of congenital coronary anomalies with multislice computed tomography. Mayo Clin Proc 2004; 79: 1017–23.
79. Lessick J, Kumar G, Beyar R et al. Anomalous origin of a posterior descending artery from the right pulmonary artery: report of a rare case diagnosed by multidetector computed tomography angiography. J Comput Assist Tomogr 2004; 28: 857–9.
80. Sato Y, Inoue F, Matsumoto N et al. Detection of anomalous origins of the coronary artery by means of multislice computed tomography. Circ J 2005; 69: 320–4.
81. Schmid M, Achenbach S, Ludwig J et al. Visualization of coronary artery anomalies by contrast-enhanced multi-detector row spiral computed tomography. Int J Cardiol 2006; 111: 430–5.
82. Roberts W, Jones AA, Nissen SE. Coronary intravascular ultrasound: implications for a quantitation of coronary arterial narrowing at necropsy in sudden coronary death. Am J Cardiol 1979; 44: 39–44.
83. Mintz GS, Painter JA, Pichard AD et al. Atherosclerosis in angiographically 'normal' coronary artery reference segments: an intravascular ultrasound study with clinical correlations. J Am Coll Cardiol 1995; 25: 1479–85.

84. Little WC, Constantinescu M, Applegate RJ et al. Can coronary angiography predict the site of a subsequent myocardial infarction in patients with mild-to-moderate coronary artery disease? Circulation 1988; 78: 1157–66.
85. Falk E, Shah PK, Fuster V. Coronary plaque disruption. Circulation 1995; 92: 657–71.
86. Leber AW, Knez A, Becker A et al. Accuracy of multidetector spiral computed tomography in identifying and differentiating the composition of coronary atherosclerotic plaques: a comparative study with intracoronary ultrasound. J Am Coll Cardiol 2004; 43: 1241–7.
87. Achenbach S, Moselewski F, Ropers D et al. Detection of calcified and noncalcified coronary atherosclerotic plaque by contrast-enhanced, submillimeter multidetector spiral computed tomography: a segment-based comparison with intravascular ultrasound. Circulation 2004; 109: 14–7.
88. Schoenhagen P, Tuzcu EM, Stillman AE et al. Non-invasive assessment of plaque morphology and remodeling in mildly stenotic coronary segments: comparison of 16-slice computed tomography and intravascular ultrasound. Coron Artery Dis 2003; 14: 459–62.
89. Schroeder S, Kopp AF, Baumbach A et al. Noninvasive detection and evaluation of atherosclerotic coronary plaques with multislice computed tomography. J Am Coll Cardiol 2001; 37: 1430–5.
90. Baumgart D, Schmermund A, Goerge G et al. Comparison of electron beam computed tomography with intracoronary ultrasound and coronary angiography for detection of coronary atherosclerosis. J Am Coll Cardiol 1997; 30: 57–64.
91. Rasouli ML, Shavelle DM, French WJ et al. Assessment of coronary plaque morphology by contrast-enhanced computed tomographic angiography: comparison with intravascular ultrasound. Coron Artery Dis 2006; 17: 359–64.
92. Budoff MJ. Prevalence of soft plaque detection with computed tomography. J Am Coll Cardiol 2006; 48: 319–21.
93. Moselewski F, Ropers D, Pohle K et al. Comparison of measurement of cross-sectional coronary atherosclerotic plaque and vessel areas by 16-slice multidetector computed tomography versus intravascular ultrasound. Am J Cardiol 2004; 94: 1294–7.
94. Di Carli MF, Dorbala S, Limaye A et al. Clinical value of hybrid PET/CT cardiac imaging: complementary roles of multi-detector CT coronary angiography and stress PET perfusion imaging. J Am Coll Cardiol 2006; 47: 115A.
95. Hacker M, Jakobs T, Matthiesen F et al. Comparison of spiral multidetector CT angiography and myocardial perfusion imaging in the noninvasive detection of functionally relevant coronary artery lesions: first clinical experiences. J Nucl Med 2005; 46: 1294–300.
96. Rispler S, Roguin A, Keidar Z et al. Integrated SPECT/CT for the assessment of hemodynamically significant coronary artery lesions. J Am Coll Cardiol 2006; 47: 115A.
97. Schuijf JD, Wijns W, Jukema JW et al. Relationship between noninvasive coronary angiography with multi-slice computed tomography and myocardial perfusion imaging. J Am Coll Cardiol 2006; 48: 2508–14.
98. Di Carli M, Hachamovitch R. New technology for noinvasive evaluation of coronary artery disease. Circulation 2007; 115: 1464–80.
99. US Food and Drug Administration, Center for Devices and Radiological Health. Whole body scanning using computed tomography (CT): what are the radiation risks from CT? Available at www.fda.gov/cdrh/ct/risks.html Accessed July 20, 2006.
100. Cohnen M, Poll L, Puttmann C et al. Radiation exposure in multi-slice CT of the heart [published correction in Rofo. 2001; 173: 521]. Rofo 2001; 178: 295–9.
101. Thomton FJ, Paulson EK, Yoshizumi TT et al. Single versus multi-detector row CT: comparison of radiation doses and dose profiles. Acad Radiol 2003; 10: 379–85.
102. Mahnken AH, Wildberger JE, Simon J et al. Detection of coronary calcifications: feasibility of dose reduction with a body weight-adapted examination protocol. AJR 2003; 181: 533–38.
103. Budoff MJ, Achenbach S, Duerinckx A. Clinical utility of computed tomography and magnetic resonance techniques for noninvasive coronary angiography. J Am Coll Cardiol 2003; 42: 1867–78.
104. Flohr TG, Schoepf UJ, Kuettner A et al. Advances in cardiac imaging with 16-section CT systems. Acad Radiol 2003; 10: 386–401.

105. Trabold T, Buchgeister M, Kuttner A et al. Estimation of radiation exposure in 16-detector row computed tomography of the heart with retrospective ECG-gating. Rofo 2003; 175: 1051–5.
106. Bae KT, Hong C, Whiting BR. Radiation dose in multidetector row computed tomography cardiac imaging. J Magn Reson Imaging 2004; 19: 859–63.
107. Raff GL, Gallagher MJ, O'Neill WW et al. Diagnostic accuracy of noninvasive coronary angiography using 64-slice spiral computed tomography. J Am Coll Cardiol 2005; 46: 552–7.
108. Gomez-Palacios M, Terron JA, Dominguez P et al. Radiation doses in the surroundings of patients undergoing nuclear medicine diagnostic studies. Health Phys. 2005; 89(2 Suppl): S27–S34
109. Picano E. Economic and biological costs of cardiac imaging. Cardiovasc Ultrasound 2005; 3: 13.
110. Poll LW, Cohnen M, Brachten S et al. Dose reduction in multi-slice CT of the heart by use of ECG-controlled tube current modulation ('ECG pulsing'): phantom measurements. Rofo 2002; 174: 1500–5.
111. Jakobs TF, Becker CR, Ohnesorge B et al. Multislice helical CT of the heart with retrospective ECG gating: reduction of radiation exposure by ECG-controlled tube current modulation. Eur Radiol 2002; 12: 1081–6.

5

Latest advances in coronary artery plaque imaging by computed tomography

Stephan Achenbach

CT technology • Coronary calcium • Coronary CTA: detection of coronary stenoses • Coronary CTA: assessment of coronary atherosclerotic plaque • Summary

Imaging of the heart and coronary arteries requires high spatial and temporal resolution. Until quite recently, computed tomography (CT) imaging did not have sufficient temporal resolution to visualize the rapidly moving heart. However, the introduction of electron beam computed tomography (EBCT) in the early 1990s and the subsequent development of multidetector CT (MDCT) scanners substantially improved the ability to perform CT imaging of cardiac structures, including the coronary arteries. EBCT imaging was initially limited to coronary calcium detection and quantification, but also allowed the first contrast-enhanced non-invasive visualization of the coronary artery lumen (coronary CT angiography, CTA).[1,2] MDCT scanners first became available in the year 2000 when 4-slice CT systems were introduced. They dramatically improved spatial resolution and overall image quality for cardiac imaging (while temporal resolution was lower than for EBCT systems). MDCT technology has been evolving rapidly – 64-slice CT systems are now widely available – and MDCT currently represents the 'gold standard' for cardiac imaging by CT. Under certain prerequisites, most prominently a low and stable heart rate, MDCT allows relatively robust visualization of the heart and coronary arteries.

Prominent recent developments have included the further evolution of CT technology, improvements in coronary CTA for stenosis detection and for visualization of coronary atherosclerotic plaque, and improvements in the clinical aspects of coronary calcium imaging for risk stratification.

CT TECHNOLOGY

The currently accepted standard for cardiac CT imaging is 64-slice CT.[3-5] The available 64-slice scanners provide rotation times between 330 and 420 ms.

With half-scan reconstruction, the temporal resolution of 64-slice CT is approximately 165 to 210 ms. So-called multisegment reconstruction algorithms can be used to improve temporal resolution by combining data sampled during several consecutive heart beats.[4] Even though the temporal resolution of CT imaging has improved substantially during the past years, it is still somewhat limited as compared to the rapid motion of the heart and especially the coronary arteries. It is currently recommended to lower the patient's heart rate to less than 60 beats/min in order to achieve optimal image quality when coronary CTA is performed with 64-slice CT equipment,[3,4] since there is a clear relationship between heart rate and image quality.[6-10] Oral or intravenous beta blockade is most often used to lower heart rate in preparation for coronary CTA, but the need to lower heart rate is frequently perceived as a major limitation of this technique.

Interestingly, while all manufacturers of CT equipment followed the same development from 4- to 16-slice CT, and now offer 64-slice scanners, they pursue different approaches to improve technology beyond 64-slice CT. One manufacturer has presented the prototype of a 256-slice system, which allows coverage of the entire heart in one single rotation.[11-13] Spatial and temporal resolution remain unchanged. This approach makes cardiac CT imaging less susceptible to arrhythmias, requires less contrast, and has the potential to reduce radiation dose.[13] Another manufacturer has made a 'dual source CT' (DSCT) system available. This system combines two X-ray tubes and detectors in a single gantry, arranged at an angular offset of 90°.[14] Only one-quarter rotation is necessary to collect the X-ray data necessary for reconstruction of an axial image and the system thus provides a temporal resolution of 83 ms, a two-fold increase in temporal resolution as compared to 64-slice CT. Initial publications demonstrate that this noticeably reduces problems caused by motion artefacts.[15-17]

CORONARY CALCIUM

In the coronary arteries, calcifications occur almost exclusively in the context of atherosclerotic changes.[18,19] The only exceptions are patients in renal failure, in whom medial (non-atherosclerotic) calcification of the coronary artery wall is thought to occur in addition to atherosclerotic calcification. Not every atherosclerotic coronary plaque is calcified, but within a coronary artery the amount of coronary calcium correlates to the extent of atherosclerotic plaque burden.[18,19] Calcification is neither a sign of stability nor instability of an individual plaque, and its presence or absence is not closely associated with the likelihood of an individual lesion to rupture and cause an event.[20] Some researchers assume calcium to be a sign of previous plaque hemorrhage, while this is disputed by others.[20] Plaques with healed ruptures usually contain calcium, whereas plaques with erosions (a less frequent mechanism of acute coronary syndromes) are often not calcified. While, therefore, the relationship between calcium and the mechanisms of acute coronary syndromes is not clearly established, the correlation of calcium with the presence and amount of coronary atherosclerotic plaque makes coronary calcium an interesting target for risk stratification purposes. In the vast majority of patients with acute coronary syndromes, some coronary calcium can be detected, and the amount of calcium in these patients is substantially greater than in matched control subjects without coronary artery disease.[21-23]

In spite of the relationship between coronary calcification and coronary plaque burden, there is only a weak correlation between the amount of coronary calcium and the angiographic severity of luminal stenosis. While even high amounts of coronary calicum do not necessarily predict the presence of coronary stenoses, the complete absence of coronary calcium makes the presence of significant luminal obstruction unlikely.[19]

Detection of coronary calcium

EBCT and MDCT with ECG gating are equally accurate for detection and quantification of coronary artery calcium[24] (Figure 5.1). Images are acquired without injection of contrast and at a relatively low radiation dose (about 0.7–3.0 mSv [25]). The amount of calcium is quantified using the so-called 'Agatston score'. Several large reference data sets are available that describe the distribution of Agatston scores found in the population, stratified by age and gender.[22,26-28] The volume and mass of calcium are alternative measures of coronary calcification, but they are not widely used even though they display a slightly better reproducibility than the Agatston score. Interscan variability for calcium quantification can be high, especially for patients with small amounts of calcium. A study in 3355 individuals found an average variability of 20% for the Agatston score and 18% for calcified plaque volume.[24]

Clinical significance of coronary calcium

Several cohort studies have shown that the presence of coronary calcium demonstrated by CT in asymptomatic individuals is a prognostic parameter with high

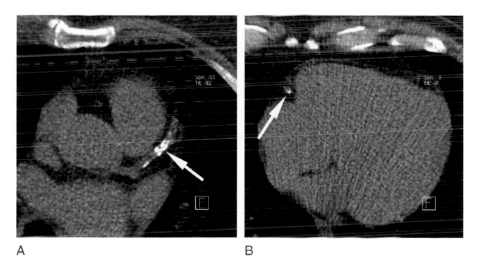

A   B

Figure 5.1   Visualization of coronary artery calcium in computed tomography. Without the injection of contrast agent, calcifications can be visualized using electron beam computed tomography (EBCT) or multidetector CT (MDCT). Here, calcifications in the left anterior descending coronary artery (A) and a small calcification in the right coronary artery (B) are visible.

predictive power regarding the development of hard cardiac events during the following 3 to 5 years.[22,29-37] A recently published meta-analysis demonstrated that a calcium score of 0 is associated with a very low risk of future myocardial infarction or death due to coronary heart disease (0.4% over 3 to 5 years).[38] The presence of any calcium increases the risk by a factor of 4. Agatston scores between 1 and 100 increase the risk of myocardial infarction and coronary artery disease death by 1.9, scores between 100 and 400 by a factor of 4.3, scores between 400 and 999 by a factor of 7.2, and scores of more than 1000 by a factor of 10.8.[38] In a recent follow-up study of 25 253 patients observed for a mean period of approximately 7 years, coronary calcium was a substantially better predictor of overall mortality than standard risk factors and the rate of death for any reason, after adjustment for traditional cardiovascular risk factors, was increased by a factor of 3.6 for Agatston scores between 11 and 100, by a factor of 3.8 for calcium scores between 101 and 399, by a factor of 5.8 for scores between 400 and 699, by a factor of 6.5 for scores between 700 and 999, and by a factor of 9.4 for scores > 1000 (see Table 5.1).[39] Interestingly, there is an influence of ethnicity both on the prevalence of coronary calcification [27] and on the predictive power of coronary calcification, with African-Americans being at highest risk when high calcum scores are present.[40]

Coronary calcification has been found to be progressive over time.[41] The amount of progression correlates to non-coronary atherosclerosis,[42] is related to cardiovascular risk factors,[43] and shows a genetic association.[44] One study has observed a higher coronary artery disease event rate in individuals who displayed more rapid progression of coronary artery calcium.[45] A number of trials have evaluated the influence of lipid-lowering therapy on the progression of coronary calcium, but they have reported conflicting results.[46-52] Currently, no sufficiently strong data are available to support the use of repeated calcium scans to guide the intensity of risk factor modification. Together with the relatively high measurement variability, especially for small amounts of calcification, this currently prevents clinical applications of repeat coronary calcium scanning.[53,54]

Table 5.1 Relationship between coronary calcium score and mortality after adjustment for cardiovascular risk factors in a cohort of 25 253 patients followed over a mean period of 6.8 ± 3 years [39]

Agatston score	Relative risk ratio (overall mortality)	Percentage of the population
0	1	44
1–10	1.48	14
11–100	3.61	20
101–399	3.84	13
400–699	5.78	4
700–999	6.47	2
>1000	9.36	4

Recommendations

In summary, coronary calcium is closely associated with coronary atherosclerosis and the predictive value of coronary calcium concerning the occurrence of future cardiovascular disease events in asymptomatic individuals is widely accepted.[38,54,55] However, it is less clear which patients or individuals will profit from having a coronary calcium scan performed. It is currently assumed that individuals clearly at high risk will not profit from coronary calcium imaging since they need intensive treatment regardless of the result:

> The current literature on coronary artery calcium does not provide support for the concept that high-risk asymptomatic individuals can safely be excluded from medical therapy for coronary heart disease even if the coronary artery calcium score is 0.

Neither will low-risk individuals profit from 'screening'.[54] Individuals who seem to be at intermediate risk for coronary events (1.0–2.0% annual risk) based on traditional risk factor analysis will be most likely to profit from coronary calcium imaging as a means of non-invasive testing for subclinical atherosclerosis in order to determine whether intensive risk modification is necessary:

> Clinical decision-making could potentially be altered by coronary artery calcium measurement in patients initially judged to be at intermediate risk (10% to 20% in 10 years). The accumulating evidence suggests that asymptomatic individuals with an intermediate Framingham Risk Score may be reasonable candidates for ... testing using coronary artery calcium as a potential means of modifying risk prediction and altering therapy.[54]

Unselected screening or patient self-referral is uniformly not recommended.[38,54,55]

CORONARY CTA: DETECTION OF CORONARY STENOSES

Improvements in scanner technology have clearly led to an improved diagnostic accuracy of CTA for the detection of coronary artery stenoses (Figures 5.2 and 5.3). A recent meta-analysis has carefully summarized the accuracy data that are available for coronary CTA,[5] and the authors demonstrated a clear increase in the accuracy for stenosis detection as scanner technology progressed from 4-slice to 16-slice and 64-slice equipment (see Table 5.2). For 64-slice CT, the pooled data indicated a sensitivity of 93% and specificity of 96% for the detection of coronary artery stenoses on a per-segment level, as well as a sensitivity of 99% and specificity of 93% based on per-patient analysis (363 patients in total). While the available data illustrate the high accuracy of coronary CTA for the detection of coronary artery stenoses, it needs to be taken into account that most studies were performed in somewhat selected patients with a rather low pretest likelihood of disease, stable sinus rhythm, ability to perfom a 10-second breathhold, and absence of renal failure. Also, studies were conducted in experienced centers, ususally with tight measures to assure a low heart rate during the scan.

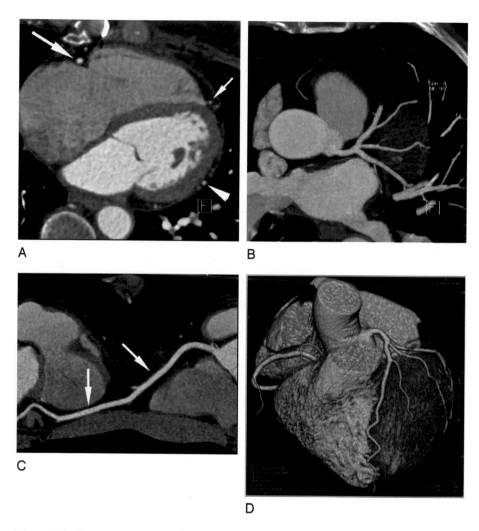

Figure 5.2 Coronary artery visualization by contrast-enhanced MDCT. (A) Transaxial image (0.75 mm slice thickness) acquired after intravenous injection of contrast agent. Cross-sections of the coronary arteries can be seen (large arrow = right coronary artery, small arrow = left anterior descending coronary artery, arrowhead = large intermediate branch). (B) In this 5-mm thick projectional image, long segments of the left main, left anterior desendding coronary artery (with a diagonal branch), ramus intermedius, and left circumflex coronary artery can be seen. (C) Curved multiplanar reconstruction which shows the entire course of the right coronary artery. (D) 3D reconstruction of the heart and coronary arteries.

Several trials have convincingly shown that high heart rates and extensive calcification negatively influence accuracy.[9,56,57] For this reason, the high accuracy values may not be generalizeable to unselected patient populations and less experienced centers. Three very recent, small trials have analyzed the diagnostic accuracy of dual-source CT for the detection of coronary artery stenoses without the use of beta-blockade to lower the heart rate. They report sensitivities of 90 to 96% and specificities of 95 to 98% for the detection of coronary stenoses with more than 50% diameter stenosis.[58–60]

Table 5.2   Meta-analysis of the sensitivity and specificity of coronary CTA with 4-, 16-, and 64-slice CT for the detection of coronary artery stenoses in comparison to invasive coronary angiography.[5]

Scanner type	Number of studies	Per-segment analysis		Per-patient analysis	
		Sensitivity (%)	Specificity (%)	Sensitivity (%)	Specificity (%)
4-slice CT	22	84	93	91	83
16-slice CT	26	83	96	97	81
64-slice CT	6	93	96	99	93

The relatively straightforward data acquisition, robust image quality, and high accuracy for the detection of coronary artery stenoses makes coronary CTA an attractive method for non-invasive evaluation of patients with suspected coronary artery disease. While it is no substitute for stress testing, because CT is unable to assess the functional relevance of a lesion, and while it is not applicable in a variety of patients, e.g. those with atrial fibrillation or renal failure, there are potential indications for its clinical use. Most prominently, CTA is able to reliably rule out coronary artery stenoses in patients who have suspected coronary artery disease, but in whom the likelihood for the presence of coronary stenoses is not very high. Table 5.3 lists potential circumstances in which CTA has been considered 'appropriate' by a US-based consensus panel of experts from various professional organizations.[61] It can be expected that future, outcome-based studies will help to better clarify the potential clinical role of CT coronary angiography in the setting of suspected coronary artery stenoses. Because of difficulties in reliably visualizing and interpreting the lumen of coronary stents by CT, and because of problems in assessing the anastomotic site of bypass grafts and the native vessels in patients after bypass surgery, the use of coronary CTA was not considered 'appropriate' in patients after coronary revascularization by stent placement or bypass surgery.[61]

CORONARY CTA: ASSESSMENT OF CORONARY ATHEROSCLEROTIC PLAQUE

Beyond the detection of coronary artery stenoses, coronary CTA is able to demonstrate coronary atherosclerotic plaque, both calcified and, if image quality

Table 5.3   'Appropriate' indications for CT coronary angiography according to an expert consensus document[61]

Detection of CAD with prior test results – Evaluation of chest pain syndrome
   Uninterpretable or equivocal stress test result (exercise, perfusion, or stress echo)
Detection of CAD: symptomatic – Evaluation of chest pain syndrome
   Intermediate pretest probability of CAD, ECG uninterpretable or unable to exercise
Detection of CAD: symptomatic – Acute chest pain
   Intermediate pretest probability of CAD, no ECG changes, and serial enzymes negative
Evaluation of coronary arteries in patients with new onset heart failure to assess etiology
Evaluation of suspected coronary anomalies

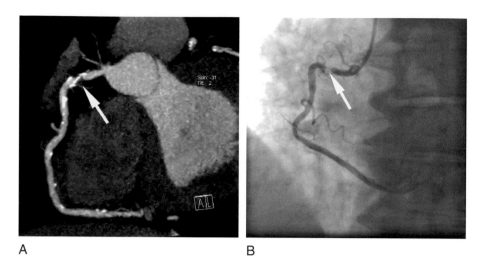

A   B

Figure 5.3 Coronary artery stenosis in contrast-enhanced coronary CT angiography. Here, a stenosis of the proximal right coronary artery is seen in CT (arrow, A) and invasive angiography (arrow, B).

is impeccable, also non-calcified (Figure 5.4). The ability to visualize non-calcified plaque components has created a lot of interest, since it is assumed that the presence of non-calcified plaque may be more predictive for future cardiovascular events than assessing calcified plaque alone. In addition, CT is thought to potentially contribute to the characterization of non-calcified plaque, in order to identify 'vulnerable' plaques at particularly high risk for rupture. These concepts are the subject of intense research, but do not currently play a clinical role.

The accuracy of coronary CTA to detect non-calcified coronary plaque is not very well known. In four small studies that compared CT to intravascular ultrasound (IVUS), sensitivities for the detection of coronary segments with plaque were reported to be approximately 80 to 90%.[62-65] Again, the data sets included in these evaluations were somewhat preselected and accuracy for plaque identification in 'real life' may be lower. Beyond detection, the characterization of coronary atherosclerotic plaque is possible to a certain extent. One parameter is the CT attenuation of the plaque material. On average, the CT attenuation within plaques classified as 'fibrous' by IVUS (and thus assumed to be relatively stable) is higher than within 'lipid-rich' plaques (mean attenuation values of 91–116 HU versus 47–71 HU).[65-70] However, the variability of density measurements within plaque types is large,[70] which currently prevents accurate classification of non-calcified 'plaque types' by coronary CTA. Other CT-based parameters that might contribute to the detection of 'vulnerable' plaques include plaque volume and the degree of remodeling; both can be assessed by CT.[65,71-73] Especially for plaque volumes measured by CT, interobserver variability has been shown to be quite high (19 to 37%).[65,74]

In spite of the astonishing ability of CT to visualize, detect, and characterize coronary atherosclerotic plaque, and the promising initial research results, there

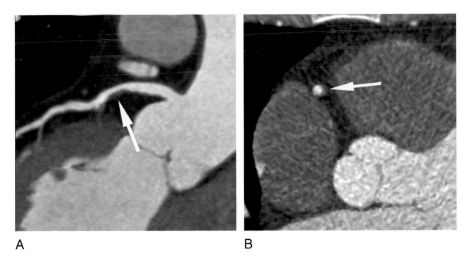

A   B

Figure 5.4 Visualization of non-calcified coronary atherosclerotic plaque in a longitudinal reconstruction of the proximal left anterior descending coronary artery (arrow, A) and in a cross-sectional view of the mid right coronary artery (arrow, B).

are currently too few clinical data to support the clinical application of contrast-enhanced coronary CTA for risk stratification purposes in asymptomatic individuals. Most of the few available studies are retrospective in nature. Four small studies have retrospectively analyzed plaque characteristics by CT in patients after acute coronary syndromes in comparison to patients with stable angina. They unanimously report a higher percentage of non-calcified plaque and more pronounced positive remodelling in lesions responsible for acute coronary events as opposed to 'stable' lesions.[75 76] A very recent analysis showed that very low CT densities measured within coronary plaques by CT (less than 30 HU) are more frequently found in lesions associated with an acute coronary syndrome.[78] The major limitation of these retrospective studies is the fact that CT data acquisition was performed *after* the acute coronary event, and thrombus formation secondary to plaque rupture may be responsibe for the appearance of these lesions in CT.

One single prospective trial concerning the predictive value of plaque seen in CT for future cardiovascular events has recently become available. Pundzuite et al followed 100 patients who underwent coronary CTA for a mean period of 16 months. They were able to demonstrate that patients with non-obstructive plaque detected by contrast-enhanced CT had a higher cardiac event rate than individuals without any plaque.[79] Most of these coronary events were 'soft' (revascularizations), and the patient numbers were extremely small, so that more data are needed before conclusions about potential clinical applications can be made.

Obviously, coronary CTA is a much more elaborate procedure than coronary calcium scanning. Radiation and contrast agent are required to obtain information about non-calcified coronary atherosclerotic plaque by CT, and it will be necessary to clearly demonstrate a substantial advantage over the analysis of traditional risk factors or other markers of atherosclerotic plaque burden (such as coronary calcium) before clinical applications of contrast-enhanced coronary CTA in asymptomatic individuals for the purpose of risk stratification can be justified. Currently, the use of coronary CTA in asymptomatic individuals for the purpose of risk stratification is discouraged.[38,61]

SUMMARY

The recent advances in scanner technology have substantially improved the ability to visualize the coronary arteries by CT. While the measurement of coronary calcium does not require the latest technology, the 'calcium score' has been convincingly demonstrated to be associated with the risk of future cardiovascular disease events and death in asymptomatic individuals. It can therefore be used in patients deemed to be at 'intermediate risk' based on traditional risk factors in order to facilitate a decision on intensive risk modification, for example the use of lipid-lowering medication.

Contrast-enhanced coronary CTA requires much higher image quality, but can be rather reliably performed with the most recent generations of CT scanners in somewhat selected patient populations. The detection of coronary artery stenoses is possible with high sensitivity and specificity and it may be clinically useful in symptomatic patients at intermediate risk for coronary artery stenoses. It has been shown that coronary CTA additionally allows for the detection and, within certain limits, the characterization of coronary atherosclerotic plaque. However, imaging is not sufficiently robust and accurate and the available clinical data are too scarce to currently allow clinical application of coronary CTA for risk stratification purposes.

REFERENCES

1. Achenbach S, Moshage W, Ropers D et al. Value of electron-beam computed tomography for the noninvasive detection of high-grade coronary-artery stenoses and occlusions. N Engl J Med 1998; 339: 1964–71.
2. Schmermund A, Rensing BJ, Sheedy PF et al. Intravenous electron-beam computed tomographic coronary angiography for segmental analysis of coronary artery stenoses. J Am Coll Cardiol 1998; 31: 1547–54.
3. Achenbach S. Cardiac CT: state of the art for the detection of coronary arterial stenosis. J Cardiovasc Comp Tomogr 2007; 1: 3–20.
4. Schoepf UJ, Zwerner PL, Savino G et al. Coronary CT angiography. Radiology 2007; 244: 48–63.
5. Vanhoenacker PK, Heijenbrok-Kal MH, Van Heste R, et al. Diagnostic performance of multidetector CT angiography for assessment of coronary artery disease: meta-analysis. Radiology 2007; 244: 419–28.
6. Leschka S, Wildermuth S, Boehm T et al. Noninvasive coronary angiography with 64-section CT: effect of average heart rate and heart rate variability on image quality. Radiology 2006; 241: 378–85.
7. Hoffmann MH, Shi H, Manzke R et al. Noninvasive coronary angiography with 16-detector row CT: effect of heart rate. Radiology 2005; 234: 86–97.
8. Herzog C, Arning-Erb M, Zangos S et al. Multi-detector row CT coronary angiography: influence of reconstruction technique and heart rate on image quality. Radiology 2006; 238: 75–86.

9. Ghostine S, Caussin C, Daoud B et al. Non-invasive detection of coronary artery disease in patients with left bundle branch block using 64-slice computed tomography. J Am Coll Cardiol 2006; 48: 1929–34.

10. Wintersperger BJ, Nikolaou K, von Ziegler F et al. Image quality, motion artifacts, and reconstruction timing of 64-slice coronary computed tomography angiography with 0.33-second rotation speed. Invest Radiol 2006; 41: 436–42.

11. Kondo C, Mori S, Endo M et al. Real-time volumetric imaging of human heart without electrocardiographic gating by 256-detector row computed tomography: initial experience. J Comput Assist Tomogr 2005; 29: 694–8.

12. Mori S, Kondo C, Suzuki N et al. Volumetric coronary angiography using the 256-detector row computed tomography scanner: comparison in vivo and in vitro with porcine models. Acta Radiol 2006; 47: 186–91.

13. Kido T, Kurata A, Higashino H et al. Cardiac imaging using 256-detector row four-dimensional CT: preliminary clinical report. Radiat Med 2007; 25: 38–44.

14. Flohr TG, McCollough CH, Bruder H et al. First performance evaluation of a dual-source CT (DSCT) system. Eur Radiol 2006; 16: 256–68.

15. Achenbach S, Ropers D, Kuettner A et al. Contrast-enhanced coronary artery visualization by dual-source computed tomography – initial experience. Eur J Radiol 2006; 57: 331–5.

16. Johnson TR, Nikolaou K, Wintersperger BJ et al. Dual-source CT cardiac imaging: initial experience. Eur Radiol 2006; 16: 1409–15.

17. Reimann AJ, Rinck D, Birinci-Aydogan A et al. Dual-source computed tomography: advances of improved temporal resolution in coronary plaque imaging. Invest Radiol 2007; 42: 196–203.

18. Burke AP, Virmani R, Galis Z et al. Task Force #2 – What is the pathologic basis for new atherosclerosis imaging techniques? J Am Coll Cardiol 2003; 41: 1874.

19. O'Rourke RA, Brundage B, Froelicher VF et al: ACC/AHA Expert Consensus Document on electron-beam computed tomography for the diagnosis and prognosis of coronary artery disease. Circulation 2000; 102: 126.

20. Pham PH, Rao DS, Vasunilashorn F et al. Computed tomography calcium quantification as a measure of atherosclerotic plaque morphology and stability. Invest Radiol 2006; 41: 674–80.

21. Pohle K, Ropers D, Mäffert R et al. Coronary calcifications in young patients with first, unheralded myocardial infarction: a risk factor matched analysis by electron beam tomography. Heart 2003; 89: 625.

22. Raggi P, Callister TQ, Cooil B et al. Identification of patients at increased risk of first unheralded acute myocardial infarction by electron-beam computed tomography. Circulation 2000; 101: 850.

23. Schmermund A, Schwartz RS, Adamzik M et al. Coronary atherosclerosis in unheralded sudden coronary death under age fifty: histopathologic comparison with 'healthy' subjects dying out of hospital. Atherosclerosis 2001; 155: 499.

24. Detrano RC, Anderson M, Nelson J et al. Coronary calcium measurements: effect of CT scanner type and calcium measure on rescan reproducibility – MESA study. Radiology 2005; 236: 477–84.

25. Gerber TC, Kuzo RS, Morin RL. Techniques and parameters for estimating radiation exposure and dose in cardiac computed tomography. Int J Cardiovasc Imaging 2005; 21: 165–76.

26. Hoff JA, Chomka EV, Krainik AJ et al. Age and gender distribution of coronary artery calcium detected by electron beam tomography in 35 246 adults. Am J Cardiol 2001; 87: 1335.

27. McClelland RL, Chung H, Detrano R et al. Distribution of coronary artery calcium by race, gender, and age. Results from the Multi-Ethnic Study of Atherosclerosis (MESA). Circulation 2006; 113; 30–37.

28. Schmermund A, Mohlenkamp S, Berenbein S et al. Population-based assesment of subclinical coronary atherosclerosis using electro-beam computed tomography. Atherosclerosis 2006; 185: 117–182.

29. Arad Y, Spadaro LA, Goodman K et al. Prediction of coronary events with electron beam computed tomography. J Am Coll Cardiol 2000; 36: 1253.

30. Park R, Detrano R, Xiang M et al. Combined use of computed tomography coronary calcium scores and C-reactive protein levels in predicting cardiovascular events in nondiabetic individuals. Circulation 2002; 106: 2073.

31. Vliegenthart R, Oudkerk M, Song B et al. Coronary calcification detected by electron-beam computed tomography and myocardial infarction. The Rotterdam Coronary Calcification Study. Eur Heart J 2002; 23: 1596.

32. Wong ND, Hsu JC, Detrano RC et al. Coronary artery calcium evaluation by electron beam computed tomography and its relation to new cardiovascular events. Am J Cardiol 2000; 86: 495.

33. Kondos GT, Hoff JA, Sevrukov A et al. Electron-beam tomography coronary artery calcium and coronary events: a 37-month follow-up of 5635 initially asymptomatic low- to intermediate-risk adults. Circulation 2003; 107: 2571.

34. Church TS, Levine BD, McGuire DK et al. Coronary artery calcium score, risk factors, and incident coronary heart disease events. Atherosclerosis 2007; 190: 224–31.

35. Taylor AJ, Bindeman J, Feuerstein I et al. Coronary calcium independently predicts incident premature coronary heart disease over measured cardiovascular risk factors: mean three-year outcomes in the Prospective Army Coronary Calcium (PACC) project. J Am Coll Cardiol 2005; 46: 807–14.

36. Greenland P, LaBree L, Azen SP et al. Coronary artery calcium score combined with Framingham score for risk prediction in asymptomatic individuals. JAMA. 2004; 291: 210–15.

37. Arad Y, Goodman KJ, Roth M et al. Coronary calcification, coronary disease risk factors, C-reactive protein, and atherosclerotic cardiovascular disease events: the St. Francis Heart Study. J Am Coll Cardiol 2005; 46: 158–65.

38. Budoff MJ, Achenbach S, Blumenthal RS et al. Assessment of coronary artery disease by cardiac computed tomography: a scientific statement from the American Heart Association Committee on Cardiovascular Imaging and Intervention, Council on Cardiovascular Radiology and Intervention, and Committee on Cardiac Imaging, Council on Clinical Cardiology. Circulation. 2006; 114: 1761–91.

39. Budoff MJ, Shaw LJ, Liu ST et al. Long-term prognosis associated with coronary calcification: observations from a registry of 25,253 patients. J Am Coll Cardiol 2007; 49: 1860–70.

40. Nasir K, Shaw LJ, Liu ST et al. Ethnic differences in the prognostic value of coronary artery calcification for all-cause mortality. J Am Coll Cardio 2007; 50: 953–60.

41. Schmermund A, Baumgart D, Möhlenkamp S et al. Natural history and topographic pattern of progression of coronary calcification in symptomatic patients. Arterioscler Thromb Vasc Biol 21: 421, 2001.

42. Taylor AJ, Bindeman J, Le TP et al. Progression of calcified coronary atherosclerosis: relationship to coronary risk factors and carotid intima-media thickness. Atherosclerosis. 2007 (Epub Ahead of Print).

43. Kronmal RA, McClelland RL, Detrano R et al. Risk factors for the progression of coronary artery calcification in asymptomatic subjects: results from the Multi-Ethnic Study of Atherosclerosis (MESA). Circulation 2007; 115: 2722–30.

44. Cassidy-Bushrow AE, Bielak LF, Sheedy PF 2nd et al. Coronary artery calcification progression is heritable. Circulation 2007; 116: 25–31.

45. Raggi P, Callister TQ, Shaw LJ. Progression of coronary artery calcium and risk of first myocardial infarction in patients receiving cholesterol-lowering therapy. Arterioscler Thromb Vasc Biol 2004; 24: 1272–7.

46. Callister TQ, Raggi P, Cooil B, et al: Effect of HmG-CoA reductase inhibitors on coronary artery disease as assessed by electron-beam computed tomography. N Engl J Med 1998; 339: 1972.

47. Achenbach S, Ropers D, Pohle K et al. Influence of lipid-lowering therapy on the progression of coronary artery calcification: a prospective evaluation. Circulation 2002; 106: 1077.

48. Budoff MJ, Lane KL, Bakhsheshi H et al. Rates of progression of coronary calcium by electron beam tomography. Am J Cardiol 2000; 86: 8.

49. Raggi P, Davidson M, Callister TQ et al. Aggressive versus moderate lipid-lowering therapy in hypercholesterolemic postmenopausal women: Beyond Endorsed Lipid Lowering with EBT Scanning (BELLES). Circulation 2005; 112: 563–71.

50. Schmermund A, Achenbach S, Budde T et al. Effect of intensive versus standard lipid-lowering treatment with atorvastatin on the progression of calcified coronary atherosclerosis over 12 months: a multicenter, randomized, double-blind trial. Circulation 2006; 113: 427–37

51. Arad Y, Spadaro LA, Roth M et al. Treatment of asymptomatic adults with elevated coronary calcium scores with atorvastatin, vitamin C, and vitamin E: the St. Francis Heart Study randomized clinical trial. J Am Coll Cardiol 2005; 46: 166–72.

52. Terry JG, Carr JJ, Kouba EO et al. Effect of simvastatin (80 mg) on coronary and abdominal aortic arterial calcium (from the coronary artery calcification treatment with zocor [CATZ] study). Am J Cardiol 2007; 99: 1714–7.

53. Taylor AJ, Bairey Merz CN, Udelson JE. 34th Bethesda Conference. Executive Summary – Can atherosclerosis imaging techniques improve the detection of patients at risk for ischemic heart disease? J Am Coll Cardiol 2003; 41: 1860.

54. Greenland P, Bonow RO, Brundage BH et al. ACCF/AHA 2007 clinical expert consensus document on coronary artery calcium scoring by computed tomography in global cardiovascular risk assessment and in evaluation of patients with chest pain: a report of the American College of Cardiology Foundation Clinical Expert Consensus Task Force (ACCF/AHA Writing Committee to Update the 2000 Expert Consensus Document on Electron Beam Computed Tomography). Circulation 2007; 115: 402–26.

55. De Backer G, Ambrosioni E, Borch-Johnsen K, et al. European guidelines on cardiovascular disease prevention in clinical practice. Third Joint Task Force of European and Other Societies on Cardiovascular Disease Prevention in Clinical Practice. Eur Heart J 2003; 24: 1601–10.

56. Grosse C, Globits S, Hergan K. Forty-slice spiral computed tomography of the coronary arteries: assessment of image quality and diagnostic accuracy in a non-selected patient population. Acta Radiol 2007; 48: 36–44.

57. Hoffmann U, Moselewski F, Cury RC et al. Predictive value of 16-slice multidetector spiral computed tomography to detect significant obstructive coronary artery disease in patients at high risk for coronary artery disease: patient versus segment-based analysis. Circulation 2004; 110: 2638–43.

58. Scheffel H, Alkadhi H, Plass A et al. Accuracy of dual-source CT coronary angiography: first experience in a high pre test probability population without heart rate control. Eur Radiol 2006; 16: 2739–47.

59. Weustink AC, Meijboom WB, Mollet NR, et al. Reliable high speed coronary computed tomography in symptomatic patients. J Am Coll Cardiol 2007; 50: 786–94.

60. Leber AW, Johnson T, Becker A, et al. Diagnostic accuracy of dual-source multi-slice CT-coronary angiography in patients with an intermediate pretest likelihood for coronary artery disease. Eur Heart J 2007; 28: 2354–60.

61. Hendel RC, Patel MR, Kramer CM et al. ACCF/ACR/SCCT/SCMR/ASNC/NASCI/SCAI/SIR 2006 appropriateness criteria for cardiac computed tomography and cardiac magnetic resonance imaging: a report of the American College of Cardiology Foundation Quality Strategic Directions Committee Appropriateness Criteria Working Group, American College of Radiology, Society of Cardiovascular Computed Tomography, Society for Cardiovascular Magnetic Resonance, American Society of Nuclear Cardiology, North American Society for Cardiac Imaging, Society for Cardiovascular Angiography and Interventions, and Society of Interventional Radiology. J Am Coll Cardiol 2006; 48: 1475–97.

62. Achenbach S, Moselewski F, Ropers D et al. Detection of calcified and noncalcified coronary atherosclerotic plaque by contrast-enhanced, submillimeter multidetector spiral computed tomography: a segment-based comparison with intravascular ultrasound. Circulation 2004; 109: 14–17.

63. Leber AW, Knez A, Becker A et al. Accuracy of multidetector spiral computed tomography in identifying and differentiating the composition of coronary atherosclerotic plaques: a comparative study with intracoronary ultrasound. J Am Coll Cardiol 2004; 43: 1241–7.

64. Schoenhagen P, Tuzcu EM, Stillman AE et al. Non-invasive assessment of plaque morphology and remodeling in mildly stenotic coronary artery segments: comparison of 16-slice computed tomography and intravascular ultrasound. Coron Artery Dis 2003; 14: 459–62.

65. Leber AW, Becker A, Knez A et al. Accuracy of 64-slice computed tomography to classify and quantify plaque volumes in the proximal coronary system: a comparative study using intravascular ultrasound. J Am Coll Cardiol 2006; 47: 672–7.

66. Schroeder S, Kopp AF, Baumbach A, et al. Noninvasive detection and evaluation of atherosclerotic coronary plaques with multislice computed tomography. J Am Coll Cardiol 2001; 37: 1430-1435.

67. Caussin C, Ohanessian A, Ghostine S, et al. Characterization of vulnerable non-stenotic plaque with 16-slice computed tomography compared with intravascular ultrasound. Am J Cardiol 2004; 94: 99-100.

68. Becker CR, Nikolaou K, Muders M, et al. Ex vivo coronary atherosclerotic plaque characterization with multi-detector-row CT. Eur Radiol 2003; 13: 2094-2098.

69. Carrascosa PM, Capunay CM, Garcia-Merletti P, et al. Characterization of coronary a therosclerotic plaques by multidetector computed tomography. Am J Cardiol 2006; 97: 598-602.

70. Pohle K, Achenbach S, MacNeill B, et al. Characterization of non-calcified coronary atherosclerotic plaque by multi-detector row CT: Comparison to IVUS. Atherosclerosis 2007; 190: 174-180.

71. Achenbach S, Ropers D, Hoffmann U, et al. Assessment of coronary remodeling in stenotic and non-stenotic coronary atherosclerotic lesions by multidetector spiral computed tomography. J Am Coll Cardiol 2004; 43: 842-847.

72. Moselewski F, Ropers D, Pohle K, et al. Comparison of measurement of cross-sectional coronary atherosclerotic plaque and vessel areas by 16-slice multidetector computed tomography versus intravascular ultrasound. Am J Cardiol 2004; 94: 1294-1297.

73. Bruining N, Roelandt JR, Palumbo A, et al. Reproducible coronary plaque quantification by multislice computed tomography. Catheter Cardiovasc Interv. 2007; 69: 857-865.

74. Pflederer T, Schmid M, Ropers D, et al. Interobserver variability of 64-slice computed tomography for the quantification of non-calcified coronary atherosclerotic plaque. Röfo 2007; 179: 953-957.

75. Leber AW, Knez A, White CW, et al. Composition of coronary atherosclerotic plaques in patients with acute myocardial infarction and stable angina pectoris determined by contrast-enhanced multislice computed tomography. Am J Cardiol 2003; 91: 714-718.

76. Inoue F, Sato Y, Matsumoto N, et al. Evaluation of plaque texture by means of multislice computed tomography in patients with acute coronary syndrome and stable angina. Circ J 2004; 68: 840-844.

77. Hoffmann U, Moselewski F, Nieman K, et al. Non-invasive assessment of plaque morphology and composition in culprit and stable lesions in acute coronary syndrome and stable lesions in stable angina by multidetector computed tomography. J Am Coll Cardiol. 2006; 47: 1655-1662.

78. Motoyama S, Kondo T, Sarai M, et al. Multislice computed tomographic characteristics of coronary lesions in acute coronary syndromes. J Am Coll Cardiol. 2007; 50: 319-326.

79. Pundzuite G, Schuijf JD, Jukema JW, et al. Prognostic value of multislice computed tomography coronary angiography in patients with known or suspected coronary artery disease. J Am Coll Cardiol 2007; 49: 62-70.

6

Vascular imaging

Steven B Feinstein

Introduction • Background • c-IMT • Arterial wall remodeling and vasa vasorum
• Case studies • Future advances: 3D imaging, IMV, vasa vasorum, and the therapeutic
uses of ultrasound • Summary of the clinical observations

INTRODUCTION

Today with the increased ingestion of diets composed of high contents of saturated
fats and carbohydrates, and sedentary lifestyle behaviors, the incidence of cardiovascular disease is expected to increase significantly associated with the prevalence
of the metabolic syndrome and type II diabetes. A recent review of the subject highlighted the worldwide epidemic.[1] Today 58 million people per year die from cardiovascular (CV) disease, with diabetes and hypertension serving as the main
predisposing factors. Nearly 1.3 billion people are considered overweight, with
312 million classified as obese, and 155 million are children by WHO definitions.
According to the authors, obesity rates have tripled in developing countries which
have achieved a Western lifestyle, and in particular the Middle East, Pacific Islands,
and South East Asia and China. With regard to diabetes, today it is estimated that
147 million people exhibit impaired glucose tolerance, which is predicted to
increase to 420 million people by 2025, and is most notable in developing countries.

Hidden within these daunting lifestyle-induced facts is the lurking danger of
insidious diseases that affect the CV system. Of particular concern, the heart and
the cerebral vascular system are targets of premature atherosclerosis. It is well
established that diabetes and the metabolic syndrome substantially increase the
morbidity and mortality of the world's populations. Therefore, the ambitious
goal of detecting preclinical disease represents a worldwide challenge.
Optimally, those individuals considered at increased risk for a CV event can be,
in part, effectively diagnosed using non-invasive, imaging technologies, leading
to subsequent aggressive treatment plans.

There are several standard population-based methologic systems used to stratify
at-risk patients. One of the most often cited is the Framingham risk profile. This
is readily available for determining one's risk profile and can be located on
the Internet.[2] The Framingham scoring system uses the following criteria as
indicators of CV disease: age, gender, smoking, cholesterol, family history of CV

disease and hypertension. Within the Framingham system, the age of the individual is heavily weighted (as an example, men between the ages of 50 and 59 have an average 10-year risk of 16%, simply based on age). With regard to generalizability of the Framingham model, the data base consisted primarily of a Caucasian, male population; thus, the applicability of the Framingham data among diverse ethnic populations has not been established.

Thus it is necessary to develop safe, non-invasive preventive measures to identify at-risk individuals who are not that is outside of the adequately characterized by the Framingham data due, perhaps, to an underestimation of the prevalence of CV disease in a population   descriptors contained within the Framingham cohort.

This chapter will review the data on using the carotid ultrasound examination of the carotid intima media thickness as a surrogate marker of premature atherosclerosis in populations that are considered to be at risk of premature cardiovascular diseases.

BACKGROUND

Recently the terms 'vulnerable' patient and 'vulnerable plaque' have been developed to identify those individuals that are at high risk of suffering an imminent CV event. By identifying individuals as vulnerable or high-risk patients, physicians and researchers worldwide have turned their focus towards attempting to identify these individuals by using non-invasive technologies. Naghavi et al have suggested that we incorporate new technologies along with the standard Framingham data base in order to characterize more completely those individuals who are at an increased risk for developing premature CV diseases.[3,4] In developing the SHAPE III guidelines, these authors have promoted and incorporated non-invasive imaging technologies (notably, c-IMT and coronary artery calcium scoring) along with traditional risk factor analyses.[5]

c-IMT

Ultrasound scanning of the carotid artery, when used to measure the c-IMT of the vessel walls, is a well-established, commonly utilized surrogate marker for atherosclerosis. Pignoli et al first described the c-IMT in 1986,[6,7] and Pagnoli's initial work has since been cited in the literature over 1000 times. Of note, using the search phase 'carotid IMT' there were 1965 listings as of 1 November, 2007 (Entrez Med search), including a recent meta-analysis of the value of using c-IMT to estimate CV risk in patients.[8]

Definitions

The ultrasound appearance of the c-IMT is based on the histopathology of the carotid artery vessel wall. The layers have been defined as follows:

(1) *Intima layer.* This layer is the first cellular layer bordering on the vessel lumen. Typically, this layer contains the luminal border-endothelial cells, foam cells, raised lesions, plaques, accompanying neovascularization and vasa vasorum, and complex luminal morphologic anatomy.

(2) *Media layer*. This is the predominant component identified using ultrasound examination of the c-IMT. The media of the arterial wall is composed of smooth muscle cells, monocytes, fibroblasts, monocyte-derived macrophages, foam cells, collagen and calcium deposition, and complex plaque formations including vasa vasorum neovascularization.

The combined intima and media layers are described as c-IMT. Similar measurements of the femoral artery have been used for atherosclerosis detection, as described by Blankenhorn et al.[9]

Validation of the c-IMT and ultrasound detection methods

The c-IMT was initially established by Pignoli et al in 1896.[7] In 1993, Wong et al performed a comparative premorbid and autopsy examination of the c-IMT in patients.[9] From this study, they demonstrated that the use of carotid ultrasound accurately identified the far wall of the common carotid artery; however, it consistently underestimated the near wall by 20%. Subsequent investigators have shown a clear correlation between the image and the anatomy and a consistent finding supporting the difficulty in identifying the near and far wall of the vessel lumen due, in part, to the physical parameters attributed to ultrasound acoustics along with the associated physical and technologic imaging limitations.[11,12]

The literature is replete with clinical trials illustrating the close association of carotid intima-media thickness (c-IMT) and the progression and regression of atherosclerosis.[8] A complete listing of the multitudes of clinical trials associated with the measurement of c-IMT is beyond the scope of this chapter, and one is referred to excellent recent reviews on the subject.[13,14]

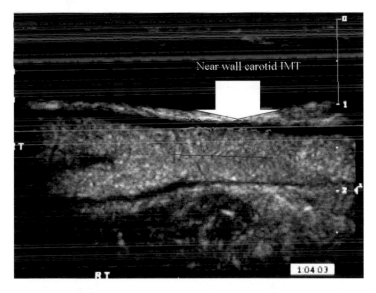

Figure 6.1 The photograph represents a longitudinal image of a contrast-enhanced, carotid artery image. The lumen is highlighted following an intravenous ultrasound contrast injection. The green dashed line represents the near wall computer-aided, contrast-enhanced, c-IMT. The outer wall, media-adventitial border, is defined by the parallel red dashed line.

In 2004 we first described the use of intravenous ultrasound contrast agents to enhance the carotid artery vessel wall lumen and highlight vessel wall luminal morphology including plaques, ulcers, and irregular luminal surfaces. In addition, we identified that the use of ultrasound contrast agents permitted an enhanced ability to detect the carotid artery IMT of the traditional, difficult to image near wall.[11] Finally, we recently published our findings in which we performed ultrasound contrast imaging in patients with significant findings of carotid artery atherosclerosis. We also reported on the direct visualization of the angiogenesis identified within atherosclerotic human plaque.[15-17] Figure 6.1 illustrates the use of contrast ultrasound to identify the near wall of the carotid artery.

ARTERIAL WALL REMODELING AND VASA VASORUM

It is postulated the initial insult to the vessel wall occurs in the endothelial layer of the artery. Additionally, the luminal turbulence[18,19] may contribute to the inuation of noxious agents due to the prolonged exposure times based on the helical flow patterns which induce wall stress at turbulant junctures (i.e., carotid bifurcation). In association with the pathologic thickening of the arterial wall the artery appears to remodel (thicken and enlarge the lumen). This remodeling appears to be a result of the vessel wall inflammation induced by the luminal infiltration initiated by noxious agents such as oxidized LDL, Lp(a) AGE products, leukocytes, monocytes, macrophages, free hemoglobin, and cytokines. The localized hypoxia and inflammation within the vessel wall institute a response which subsequently signals the production of the VEGF family of proteins and leads to the growth of neovascularization throughout the vessel wall. Remodeling of the carotid artery, initially described by Glagov et al in 1993,[19] was observed in Figure 6.2.

In 2003 we were the first to observe the presence of the carotid arterial vasa vasorum in patients with cerebral vascular disease, as noted in Figure 6.3.[16] In this particular clinical situation, the patient did not experience symptomatic cerebral vascular disease. Yet, remarkably, the intra-arterial wall vasa vasorum was clearly identified following the intravenous injection of an ultrasound contrast agent (Optison, GE Health Care, Milwaukee, Wisconsin). Subsequent clinical histopathology validation studies have been performed and the results have been published by Shah et al.[20,21] Using MRI technology, the presence of angiogenesis within the arterial wall atherosclerotic plaque has been similarly identified.[22]

Based on the seminal experimental studies of Heistad, Mouten, and Wilson,[23-25] the presence of intra-arterial wall angiogenesis (vasa vasorum) appears to precede the thickening of the IMT. Of note, in 1985, Heisted demonstrated that the vasa vasorum regressed following the withdrawal of an inflammatory noxious stimulus (cholesterol feeding in primates).[22] Similarly, Wilson in 2002,[25] induced vasa vasorum regression following the use of statins in swine fed high-cholesterol diets. Using experimental models, the authors have shown that the earliest manifestation of atherosclerosis may be the presence of the arterial vasa vasorum. Fleiner et al[26] and Moreno et al,[27] through pathology studies, have linked plaque angiogenesis and plaque vulnerability.

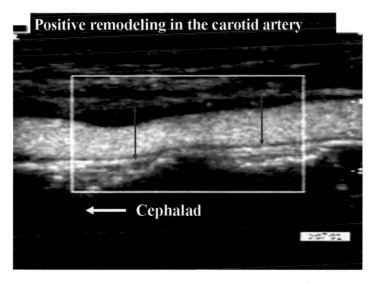

Figure 6.2 The carotid artery as presented from this photograph revealed the natural remodeling associated with the "Glagov" phenomena. Note the longitudinal view of the carotid artery lumen is highlighted following an intravenous injection of contrast (the proximal region is the right with the distal, cephalad aspect to the left). The red arrows identify the "increase" or remodeling of the luminal diameter associated with advanced atherosclerosis (also known as the "Glagov phenomena").

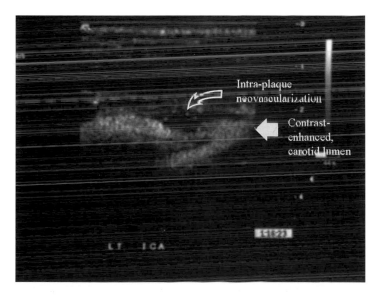

Figure 6.3 The first image of carotid plaque revascularization as identified following the use of ultrasound contrast agents. Note the intense lumen intensity and the small intra-plaque microvascular channels noted by the presence of contrast material within the intra-luminal plaque.

Historically, the observed connection between tumor growth and the vasa vasorum was proposed by Judah Folkman in 1971.[28] Folkman and Moulten et al[29] also proposed that atherosclerosis, in a manner similar to cancer tumor growth, stimulates the growth of angiogenesis, and the development of vasa vasorum.

Overall, the novel observation of detecting the presence of angiogenesis within the human atherosclerotic plaque using contrast ultrasound methods was considered a highlight in 2006 according to the editors of the Journal of the American College of Cardiology (editor, Anthony DeMaria).[30]

CASE STUDIES

Case 1

Mr L presented to our clinic for a second opinion regarding his medical and surgical evaluation of a recent, transient ischemic attack (TIA) involving numbness and tingling of his left hand. From his history, he denied prior CV disease (no past history of myocardial infarction (MI) or cerebral vascular accident (CVA)), he denied a past history of smoking, hypertension, DM, or early CV deaths in the family. His physical examination was unremarkable for lateralizing signs of a CVA. Laboratory testing revealed an elevated HgbA1C at 6.4 (normal range 3.9–6.2), the fasting blood glucose was elevated at 110 mg/dl, and the fractionated cholesterol patterns revealed a type B pattern consistent with a predominance of small dense LDL particles. The results of his ultrasound carotid examination revealed a 30–40% stenosis in the right internal carotid artery and a >75% stenosis in the left internal carotid artery. Of particular note, the patient's contrast-enhanced, ultrasound examination of his carotid artery revealed significant intraplaque neovascularization in both the right and left internal carotid arteries. Figure 6.4 reveals a still frame ultrasound image emblematic of his bilateral atherosclerosis as highlighted following the intravenous injection of ultrasound contrast agent. The treatment plan consisted of medical and surgical therapies. Subsequent to surgery, which consisted of a left carotid endarterectomy, the patient was started on medical therapy which included statins, niacin, aspirin, and a peroxisome proliferator-activated receptor (PPAR) (Pioglitazone, Takeda Pharmaceutics). Subsequently, the patient has not experienced further symptoms of a TIA, CVA, or angina, and he remains physically active.

Case 2

Mr H, a 72 year old man with no prior history of MI, CVA, diabetes, hypertension or smoking, appeared to be a well-developed, well-nourished man. His CV examination was within normal limits. However, due to complaints of visual disturbances a contrast-enhanced, carotid ultrasound examination was performed. The results indicated a >75% stenosis on the internal carotid artery with evidence of neovascularization within the atheromatous plaque (Figure 6.5). Consequently, he was referred for a surgical carotid endarterectomy. The carotid plaque histology revealed significant neovascularization within the plaque, consistent with the presurgical evaluation following the contrast-enhanced

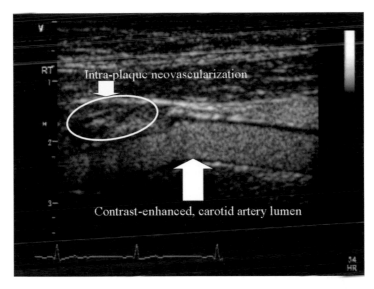

Figure 6.4 A representative image of a highly vascular carotid artery plaque as identified using ultrasound contrast imaging techniques. This patient had bilateral carotid plaques with significant neovascularization. The patient had unilateral symptoms despite bilateral disease.

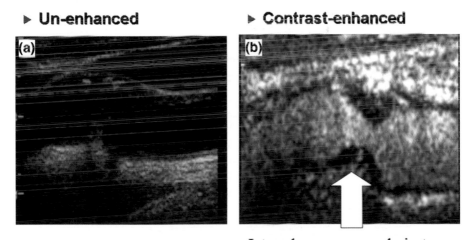

Figure 6.5 (a and b) These still frames represent the ultrasound images from a patient with severe carotid artery stenosis. (a) is the image without ultrasound contrast, (b) with ultrasound contrast enhancement. Note the presence of the microvessels within the plaques located on the near and far walls. The patient was asymptomatic with regard to cerebrovascular disease.

carotid ultrasound findings. The presence of these angiogenic adventitial vessels has been well described at the time of surgery, as noted by cardiovascular surgeons over the years (Dr Marshall Goldin, personal communication).

At follow up the patient remained in good health and he has not developed untoward symptoms of TIA, CVA, or angina pectoris.

Case 3

Mr W presented to our institution approximately 10 years ago with an acute MI. He has not experienced a subsequent MI nor a CVA or TIA. The patient had a history of hypertension and elevated cholesterol. He has been managed aggressively with medical therapy for the last 10 years.

Our contrast-enhanced carotid ultrasound examination revealed a non-obstructive carotid lesion notable for an ulcerative lesion associated with significant intraplaque neovascularization along the adventitial near wall (Figure 6.6). The patient continues to be free from CV events and is under aggressive medical management.

FUTURE ADVANCES: 3D IMAGING, INTIMA-MEDIA-VOLUME (IMV), VASA VASORUM AND THE THERAPEUTIC USES OF ULTRASOUND[16]

It is anticipated that the growing use of 3D/4D technology will be incorporated into vascular imaging in order to provide a truly volumetric analysis of the

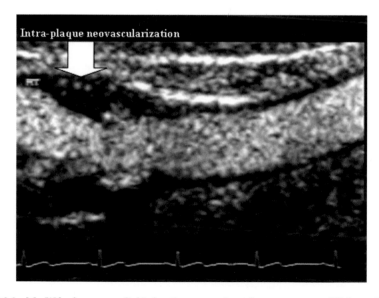

Figure 6.6   Mr. W had a myocardial infarction approximately ten years ago. While undergoing routine cardiovascular screening, he was noted to have a unilateral carotid stenosis associated with a luminal ulcer and significant intra-plaque neovascularization.

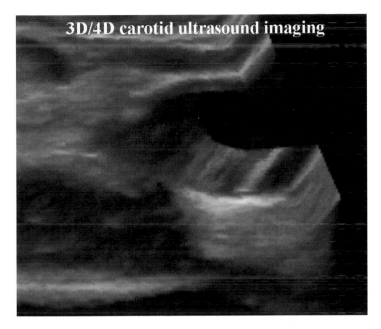

Figure 6.7 A representative sample of a real-time, volumetric display of a 3-D/4-D carotid ultrasound permitting a true volumetric analysis of the IMV.

c-IMT, improved plaque morphology, and quantitative assessment of the vasa vasorum. Our initial attempts to perform these examinations can be seen in Figure 6.7.

SUMMARY OF THE CLINICAL OBSERVATIONS

The three clinical cases presented in this chapter reveal the wide range of angiogenesis found within human carotid atherosclerotic plaques. The use of contrast-enhanced carotid ultrasound imaging provides a unique window through which we can directly view the presence of neovascularization (vasa vasorum) in individuals with both asymptomatic and symptomatic atherosclerosis. Certainly, these initial novel observations are not a substitute for large-scale, prospective clinical trials; however, they remain consistent with the experimental findings observed in animal models of atherosclerosis, particularly in those plaques that would be considered 'unstable' or 'vulnerable.' Perhaps the simple application of a contrast-enhanced ultrasound examination of the human carotid artery will provide valuable insight into the world of preclinical atherosclerosis diagnosis and treatment.

REFERENCES

1. Hossain P, Kawar B, El Nahas M. Obesity and diabetes in the developing world – a growing challenge. N Engl J Med 2007; 356(3): 213–15.
2. http://hinnihlbigov/atpiii/calculatorasap 2006.

3. Naghavi M, Libby P, Falk E et al. From vulnerable plaque to vulnerable patient: a call for new definitions and risk assessment strategies: Part I. Circulation 2003; 108(14): 1664–72.
4. Naghavi M, Libby P, Falk E et al. From vulnerable plaque to vulnerable patient: a call for new definitions and risk assessment strategies: Part II. Circulation 2003; 108(15): 1772–8.
5. Naghavi M, Falk E, Hecht HS et al. From vulnerable plaque to vulnerable patient – Part III: Executive summary of the Screening for Heart Attack Prevention and Education (SHAPE) Task Force report. Am J Cardiol 2006; 98(2A): 2–15H.
6. Pignoli P, Longo T. Ultrasound evaluation of atherosclerosis. Methodological problems and technological developments. Eur Surg Res 1986; 18(3–4): 238–53.
7. Pignoli P, Tremoli E, Poli A et al. Intimal plus medial thickness of the arterial wall: a direct measurement with ultrasound imaging. Circulation 1986; 74(6): 1399–406.
8. Lorenz MW, Markus HS, Bots ML et al. Prediction of clinical cardiovascular events with carotid intima-media thickness: a systematic review and meta-analysis. Circulation 2007; 115(4): 459–67.
9. Blankenhorn DH, Johnson RL, Nessim SA et al. The Cholesterol Lowering Atherosclerosis Study (CLAS): design, methods, and baseline results. Control Clin Trials 1987; 8(4): 356–87.
10. Wong M, Edelstein J, Wollman J et al. Ultrasonic–pathological comparison of the human arterial wall. Verification of intima-media thickness. Arterioscler Thromb 1993; 13(4): 482–6.
11. van Swijndregt ADM. An in-vitro evaluation of the line pattern of the near and far walls of carotid arteries using B-mode ultrasound. Ultrasound Med Biol 1996; 22(8): 1007–15.
12. Montauban van Swijndregt AD, De Lange EE, De Groot E et al. An in vivo evaluation of the reproducibility of intima-media thickness measurements of the carotid artery segments using B-mode ultrasound. Ultrasound Med Biol 1999; 25(3): 323–30.
13. Rajaram V, Pandhya S, Patel S et al. Role of surrogate markers in assessing patients with diabetes mellitus and the metabolic syndrome and in evaluating lipid-lowering therapy. Am J Cardiol 2004; 93(11A): 32C–48C.
14. Patel SN, Rajaram V, Pandya S et al. Emerging, noninvasive surrogate markers of atherosclerosis. Curr Atheroscler Rep 2004; 6(1): 60–8.
15. Macioch JE, Katsamakis CD, Robin J et al. Effect of contrast enhancement on measurement of carotid artery intimal medial thickness. Vasc Med 2004; 9(1): 7–12.
16. Feinstein SB. The powerful microbubble: from bench to bedside, from intravascular indicator to therapeutic delivery system, and beyond. Am J Physiol Heart Circ Physiol 2004; 287(2): H450–7.
17. Feinstein SB. Contrast ultrasound imaging of the carotid artery vasa vasorum and atherosclerotic plaque neovascularization. J Am Coll Cardiol 2006; 48(2): 236–43.
18. Morbiducci U, Ponzini R, Grigioni M et al. Helical flow as fluid dynamic signature for atherogenesis risk in aortocoronary bypass. A numeric study. J Biomech 2007; 40(3): 519–34.
19. Glagov S, Zarins CK, Masawa N et al. Mechanical functional role of non-atherosclerotic intimal thickening. Front Med Biol Eng 1993; 5(1): 37–43.
20. Neems R FM, Goldin M, Dainauskas J et al. Real-time contrast enhanced ultrasound imaging of neovascularization within the human carotid plaque. J Am Col Cardiol 2004; 43(5): 374A.
21. Shah F, Balan P, Weinberg M et al. Contrast enhanced ultrasound imaging of atherosclerotic carotid plaque neovascularization – a new surrogate marker of atherosclerosis? J Vasc Med 2007; 12(4): 291–7.
22. Kerwin W, Hooker A, Spilker M et al. Quantitative magnetic resonance imaging analysis of neovasculature volume in carotid atherosclerotic plaque. Circulation 2003; 107(6): 851–6.
23. Heistad DD, Armstrong ML. Blood flow through vasa vasorum of coronary arteries in atherosclerotic monkeys. Arteriosclerosis 1986; 6(3): 326–31.
24. Moulton KS. Plaque angiogenesis and atherosclerosis. Curr Atheroscler Rep 2001; 3(3): 225–33.
25. Wilson SH, Herrmann J, Lerman LO et al. Simvastatin preserves the structure of coronary adventitial vasa vasorum in experimental hypercholesterolemia independent of lipid lowering. Circulation 2002; 105(4): 415–8.
26. Fleiner M, Kummer M, Mirlacher M et al. Arterial neovascularization and inflammation in vulnerable patients: early and late signs of symptomatic atherosclerosis. Circulation 2004; 110(18): 2843–50.

27. Moreno PR, Purushothaman KR, Fuster V et al. Plaque neovascularization is increased in ruptured atherosclerotic lesions of human aorta: implications for plaque vulnerability. Circulation 2004; 110(14): 2032–8.
28. Folkman J. Tumor angiogenesis: therapeutic implications. N Engl J Med 1971; 285(21): 1182–6.
29. Moulton KS, Vakili K, Zurakowski D et al. Inhibition of plaque neovascularization reduces macrophage accumulation and progression of advanced atherosclerosis. Proc Natl Acad Sci USA 2003; 100(8): 4736–41.
30. DeMaria AN, Ben-Yehuda O, Feld GK et al. Highlights of the year in JACC 2006. J Am Coll Cardiol 2007; 49(4): 509–27.

7

Surrogate markers in atherosclerosis

Michael H Davidson

Treatment of emerging risk factors • Non-invasive tests for preclinical disease

TREATMENT OF EMERGING RISK FACTORS

Lipoprotein(a)

Lipoprotein(a) (Lp(a)) is a low-density lipoprotein (LDL) particle with an apolipoprotein apo(a) attached. Apo(a) is linked to LDL by a disulfide bond with a repeating kringle structure (named for a looped Scandinavian pastry) (Figure 7.1),[1] This structure has significant homology to plasminogen, and the enhanced coronary heart disease (CHD) risk associated with Lp(a) is reportedly due to the inhibiting effects of this lipoprotein particle on plasminogen activation, leading to enhanced thrombosis. Lp(a) may also increase the atherogenicity of LDL.[2-4] The majority of observational trials (10 of 15) support the association of Lp(a) with enhanced cardiovascular risk. Every 30 mg per dL increase in Lp(a) approximately doubles the risk of CHD. The distribution of Lp(a) levels in the population is different from the bell-shaped curve for serum cholesterol, but the majority of Americans have low levels (less than 10 mg/dl), with a small percentage having greater than 30 mg/dl.[5] Elevated Lp(a) is more common in the Asian Indian and Turkish populations.

Therapeutical modification of Lp(a) is controversial, and only two pharmacologic treatments, niacin and estrogen, modestly lower Lp(a).[6] Both niacin and estrogen lower Lp(a) by approximately 20%. A post hoc analysis of the Heart and Estrogen/Progestin Replacement Study demonstrated that for women with CHD with the highest quartile of Lp(a), HRT resulted in a significant reduction in subsequent coronary events. In the Familial Atherosclerosis Treatment Study, the lowering of Lp(a) with niacin appeared to beneficially modify atherosclerotic progression as determined by quantitative angiography.[7] These trials are supportive, but not conclusive, that lowering Lp(a) with either estrogen or niacin may be beneficial. Another approach for the patient with elevated Lp(a) is to significantly lower LDL. Transgenic mice expressing human Apo(a) developed vascular lesions only when fed a lipid-rich diet, not when fed normal chow. In addition, the odds ratio for having significant angiographic CHD in patients with high (greater than 30 mg/dl) versus low (less than or equal to 5 mg/dl)

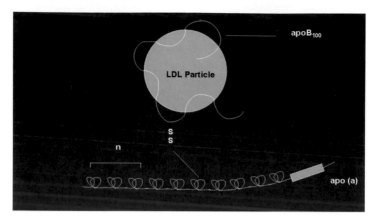

Figure 7.1   Structure of Lipoprotein(a). (Adapted from seed et al J Cardiovasc Risk 1995; 2: 206–15)

Lp(a) levels increased from 1.67 to 6.0, as concomitant LDL concentrations increased.[8-9] Therefore, Lp(a) may be a significantly less important risk factor if LDL is less than 100 mg/dl. If Lp(a) is elevated and treatment is deemed necessary in the judgment of the physician, the decision to use niacin or estrogen for women is enhanced, but the primary focus of therapy should be to aggressively lower LDL or non-high density lipoprotein (HDL) to the appropriate goals.[10]

Homocysteine

Homocysteine is an amino acid that, if elevated, results in an increased risk of CHD. The strength of this association is debatable, but, clearly, patients with an inherited defect in homocysteine catabolism resulting in hyperhomocysteinuria have a markedly increased risk of premature atherosclerosis and thrombosis.[11] These rare genetic deficiencies of either methylenetetrahydrofolate reductase or of cobalamin metabolism result in homocysteinuria in which 30% of untreated patients have thrombotic events by age 20 years. These genetic enzyme deficiencies are rare, but many other factors may affect homocysteine levels. The most important acquired causes of increased homocysteine levels are nutritional deficiency of either folate, vitamin B_{12}, or vitamin B_6. Because homocysteine levels can be effectively lowered with vitamin supplementation, this risk factor is an intriguing target for therapeutic intervention.[12-13] A meta-analysis of both retrospective and prospective trials demonstrated a moderate but relatively consistent association between homocysteine and increased CHD and cerebrovascular events. Because factors that raise homocysteine, such as a folate-deficient diet (low in green vegetables), hypothyroidism, and renal failure, may be independently associated with increased CHD risk, the value of measuring and treating high homocysteine levels is uncertain. Furthermore, after the fortification of the US food supply with folate to reduce the incidence of neural tube birth defects, the number of patients with moderate hyperhomocysteinemia is likely to be small. Therefore, neither the American College of Cardiology nor the American Heart Association advocates population-based screening for homocysteine. In addition, due to the high cost of measuring homocysteine and the relatively low cost of folate (the cost of one homocysteine blood test is approximately equivalent to at least 2 years of folate therapy), many experts advocate folate, B_{12}, and B_6 supplementation but not routine homocysteine measurements for patients with or at high risk for CHD. There is also a lack of proven clinical trial evidence that lowering homocysteine levels with folate and other B vitamin supplementation results in reduced ischemic events. There are several ongoing vitamin trials that are prospectively evaluating the benefits of homocysteine reduction on CHD risk. Although there is no clear consensus on whom to test or treat for elevated homocysteine, in patients with premature or a strong family history for CHD or recurrent CHD with a relatively benign lipid profile, measuring homocysteine may provide useful guidance in a comprehensive risk management strategy.[12] A normal homocysteine level is less than 10 µmol/l, and, similar to serum cholesterol, the risk for CHD increases in a relatively linear manner for homocysteine levels between 10 and 15 µmol/l. If homocysteine is elevated, often a multivitamin with 400 mg of folate is sufficient to lower the level to normal, but certain patients require higher doses of folate or other factors that enhance homocysteine catabolism to satisfactorily lower the level to below 10 µmol/l. However, several recent trials have demonstrated that folic acid supplementation does not affect coronary outcomes.

C-reactive protein

C-reactive protein (CRP) is a marker of general inflammation reflecting the formation of foam cells formed from macrophages engulfing oxidized LDL particles. Foam cells secrete interleukin-6 that induces the liver to secrete CRP. CRP is the best studied of a series of inflammatory markers that appear to predict CHD risk. The concentration of CRP associated with atherosclerosis is substantially below those of most routine CRP assays (3 mg/l), and, thus, a more sensitive assay termed *high sensitivity CRP* (hs-CRP) has been developed.[14] Several studies suggest that measurement of CRP may provide a useful method of assessing the risk of CHD in apparently healthy people, particularly when LDL is low.[15-18] In addition, the endpoint trials (Air Force/Texas Coronary Atherosclerosis Prevention Study (AF/CAPS) and Cholesterol and Recurrent Events) have demonstrated that statins lower CRP and that this reduction of CRP is associated with a reduction in endpoints, but this effect of statin may be independent of its effect on cholesterol. All statins appear to lower CRP. In a cross-over study, with equal lowering of LDL, atorvastatin, simvastatin, and pravastatin lowered CRP equally. There appears to be a greater difference in that, in apparently healthy women, CRP levels greater than 1.5 mg/l predict 3 to 7 times the risk for MI or stroke, but for men, a CRP level greater than 2.11 mg/l predicts 3 times the risk for MI and 2 times the risk for ischemic stroke; There also appears to be a lag time between the detection of elevated CRP and when an atherosclerotic event occurs. The test is most predictive for risk of an event 4 to 6 years later. CRP as a risk predictor alone is comparable to the total cholesterol to HDL ratio and is additive to the ratio when used in combination.

The more criteria for the metabolic syndrome the patient has, the more likely CRP will be elevated. However, even for those patients with the metabolic syndrome, the presence of an elevated CRP is associated with an increased risk of CHD. In the AFCAPS/TexCAPS trial,[19] a post hoc analysis demonstrated that patients with an LDL below the median but a CRP above the median had the same relative risk reduction on statin therapy as those with high LDL. The hypothesis that patients with elevated CRP levels but LDL levels that are below the National Cholesterol Education Program (NCEP)[20] ATP III drug treatment initiation thresholds will benefit from lipid-lowering therapy is being tested in the ongoing Justification for Use of statins in Primary prevention: an Intervention Trial Evaluating Rosuvastatin.[21] This is a randomized trial of 15 000 patients with a CRP level greater than 2.0 mg/dl but an LDL level less than 130 mg/dl treated with rosuvastatin, 20 mg/l, or with placebo. Besides statins, other lipid-lowering agents, such as niacin, fibrates, and ezetimibe, have been shown to lower CRP levels. According to the AHA/Centers for Disease Control Scientific Statement on Markers of Intervention and Cardiovascular Disease, the patient with an intermediate Framingham ATP III 10-year risk score of 10 to 20% with an LDL level below the cutpoint for initiation of drug therapy is the most appropriate patient in whom to measure CRP level (Figure 7.2).[22-23] The basis for this recommendation is that in this intermediate risk group, an elevated CRP level would provide a rationale to initiate lipid-lowering therapy. In patients already known to be at high risk, such as those with diabetes, CHD, or a greater than 20% Framingham 10-year risk score, measuring CRP level would not be necessary because the initiation of lipid-lowering therapy is clearly indicated. The AHA/Centers for Disease Control panel considered recommending more widespread testing of CRP level, such as in those patients with a family history of CHD or the metabolic syndrome, but considered the evidence inadequate at this time. For patients with CHD, more aggressive treatment of LDL in those with an elevated CRP has not yet been demonstrated to be beneficial in clinical

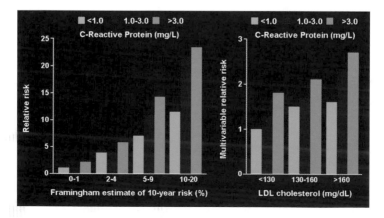

Figure 7.2   CRP adds prognostic information at all levels of LDL-c and at all levels of the Framingham risk score. (Adapted from Ridker et al[18])

trials. As more evidence accumulates regarding the benefits of CRP testing, the recommendation as to which patients are likely to benefit from testing is likely to broaden.

Lipoprotein-associated phospholipase A2

Lipoprotein-associated phospholipase A2 (Lp-PLA$_2$) is a subtype of the phospholipase A2 superfamily, a family of enzymes that hydrolyze phospholipids. Lp-PLA2, also known as *platelet-activating factor acetylhydrolase*, is a 50-kD, Ca^{2+}-independent phospholipase that is distinct from another macrophage product, secretary PLA2, a 14-kD, Ca-dependent enzyme. Increasing evidence suggests that Lp-PLA$_2$ plays a critical role in the vascular inflammatory process that leads to the development of atherosclerosis and its clinical sequelae.[24] Lp-PLA$_2$ activity is upregulated in atherosclerotic plaques and, when released into circulation, binds specifically to LDL. The key role of Lp-PLA$_2$ in atherogenesis is its hydrolysis of oxidized LDL, which is generated when LDL becomes oxidized in the milieu of the artery wall. The hydrolysis of oxidized LDL by Lp-PLA$_2$ produces the proinflammatory, atherogenic byproducts lysophosphatidylcholine and oxidized fatty acids. Lysophosphatidylcholine plays a critical role in atherogenesis. It acts as a chemoattractant for monocytes, impairs endothelial function, causes cell death by disrupting plasma membranes, and induces apoptosis in smooth muscle cells and macrophages. Based on clinical data obtained from a number of recent epidemiologic studies, it appears that the determination of Lp-PLA$_2$ levels may aid in the identification of individuals at high risk for CHD and stroke. Elevated levels of Lp-PLA$_2$ have been shown to indicate a greater risk of plaque formation and rupture independent of traditional risk factors and CRP (Figure 7.3).[25-33] The PLAC™ test is an enzyme immunoassay developed for the quantitative determination of Lp-PLA$_2$ in human plasma to be used in conjunction with clinical evaluation and patient risk assessment in predicting risk for

Study – hard CV endpoint	Year	Population	#Cases/ #controls	Hazard ratio (for top quantile)	Relative risk (per std deviation)
WOSCOPS – coronary events	2000	Hypercholesterolemic men	580/1160	1.8	1.18
WHS – coronary events	2001	Healthy women	123/123		1.17*
ARIC – coronary events	2004	Healthy subjects LDL < 130	608/740 203/507	1.15* 2.08	
MONICA – coronary events	2004	Healthy men	97/837		1.21
ROTTERDAM – coronary events	2005	Elderly subjects	308/1820	1.97	
PROSPER – coronary events	2006	Elderly subjects	856/1801	1.25	
CHS – MI	2006	Elderly subjects	504/4318	1.26	
Rancho Bernardo – CHD events	2006	Healthy subjects	1077	1.64	
Malmo – MI and stroke	2007	MI and stroke	262	1.54	1.16

*Non-significant.

Figure 7.3 Elevated Lp-PLA2 as a predictor of coronary events in primary prevention.

CHD. Results are reliable and reproducible when the assay procedure is carried out with adherence to good laboratory practice.

Lipoprotein subfractions

Many lipid specialists use advanced laboratory testing to determine subfractions of LDL, HDL, and very-low-density lipoprotein (VLDL). The three most popular technologies that have been developed by commercial laboratories are ultracentrifugation (Berkeley Heart Labs, Berkeley, CA), vertical autoprofile (Atherotec, Birmingham, AL), and nuclear magnetic resonance (NMR) (LipoMed, Raleigh, NC). The price for the lipoprotein subfraction tests ranges from $75 to $300. The main purpose of these tests is to identify patients at higher risk for CHD due to small, dense LDL or pattern B. These tests also determine VLDL and HDL subfractions. Generally, patients with high triglyceride (TG) and low HDL have dense LDL, but between TG levels of 100 and 200 mg/dl, the likelihood of pattern B varies significantly. In the presence of hypertriglyceridemia, LDL particles are TG enriched and relatively cholesterol poor and are catalyzed by cholesterol ester transfer protein. The TG-enriched LDL particles are further degraded by hepatic lipase to form a small, dense, more atherogenic LDL particle (Figure 7.4).[34] Therefore, the total LDL level may be normal, but the number of LDL particles is significantly increased. The Quebec Cardiovascular Study followed 2000 men over a 5-year period.[35] This study demonstrated that the denser the LDL particle, the greater the increased risk for CHD, and the risk was extremely high (odds ratio of 6.2) if both the LDL particles were small and the particle concentration was high (LDL greater than 120 mg/dl). Subfactoration of VLDL and HDL has also demonstrated differences in CHD risk. Increased large VLDL particles in testing plasma correlate with impaired rates of chylomicron clearance, which

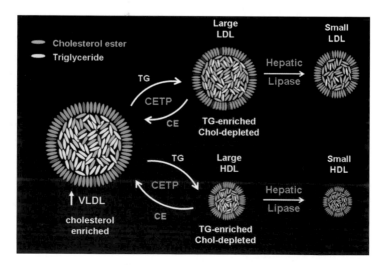

Figure 7.4   Cholesterol Carried inside Lipoprotein Particles is highly variable. (Adapted from Otvos et al[34])

independently predict CHD risk. For HDL, the larger subclasses appear to confer most of the protection from CHD, compared to the smaller HDL particles. The NMR LipoProfile determines all the various lipoprotein subclasses. The basic question regarding advanced lipoprotein testing is whether these tests should be used routinely. Because non-HDL incorporates all of the potentially atherogenic lipoproteins, perhaps simply targeting non-HDL as recommended by ATP III in patients with TG greater than 200 mg/dl is sufficient to reduce CHD risk. The superiority of lipoprotein subclass testing over non-HDL to further reduce CHD risk requires further investigation. In patients with premature CHD or a strong family history of CHD with a relatively benign lipid profile, these tests may provide the greatest value. The most promising advanced lipoprotein test is the LDL particle concentration, which determines the total number of LDL particles (nmol/l) in the blood determined by direct measurement of four LDL subclasses, including intermediate density lipoprotein (IDL). LDL particle concentration may be more strongly linked with CHD risk than LDL cholesterol and, therefore, may be a better target of therapy. Fibrates or niacin may more likely convert a patient from pattern B (dense LDL) to pattern A (large LDL) by lowering TG more than a statin, but statins are more effective at lowering LDL particle concentrations. The results of advanced lipid testing often lead to the use of combination therapy or higher dose statins to achieve the optimal targets for all the lipoprotein subclasses. Proponents of these tests believe that ultimately CHD risk assessment will be better defined and targeted treatment will more successfully prevent atherosclerosis progression. This hypothesis requires further clinical evaluation.

NONINVASIVE TESTS FOR PRECLINICAL DISEASE

The ability of traditional risk factors to predict the development of clinical atherosclerosis is, at best, 80% accurate. Advocates of non-invasive tests to evaluate the severity of preclinical atherosclerotic plaque maintain that these tests indicate the actual presence of disease rather than risk factors to disease and are, therefore, better predictors of CHD events. In addition, improvement in these surrogate markers of atherosclerosis may better indicate the benefits of therapy, or a lack of a beneficial change in these markers may mean more aggressive therapeutic interventions are necessary. The National Institutes of Health has initiated the Multi-Ethnic Study of Atherosclerosis to determine if the non-invasive assessment of preclinical disease improves risk predictability and provides clinical value beyond the traditional risk assessment scores.

One of the easiest to perform and least costly non-invasive measures of preclinical atherosclerosis is the ankle-brachial index (ABI). This test shows goal reproducibility, with 95% confidence variability of a single measurement being approximately 16%.[36-37] An ABI of less than 0.90 is commonly used as a cutpoint to define peripheral vascular disease. The NCEP ATP III also defines peripheral vascular disease as an ABI of less than 0.90, and, therefore, the LDL goal for these patients is less than 100 mg/dl. The severity of the ABI abnormality predicts cardiovascular disease mortality, and for each risk factor, the coexistence of an ABI less than 0.90 significantly increases the CHD mortality. Although ABI abnormalities increase sharply with age, for adults between the ages of 40 and 59 years only 2 to 3% have an abnormal ABI. Therefore, the ABI is a helpful screening tool to identify high-risk individuals for CHD. ABI should probably be conducted routinely on smokers older than age 40 years, because although their NCEP ATP III Framingham risk score may not be 20% or greater, an ABI of less than 0.90 would automatically place the patient in the CHD risk-equivalent category with an LDL goal of less than 100 mg/dl. In addition, these patients should be on aspirin or other antiplatelet therapy and, based on the Heart Outcomes Prevention Evaluation (HOPE) trial, may benefit from ACE inhibitors, such as ramipril, used in this trial.[38]

Carotid ultrasound has been extensively evaluated as a tool to assess CHD risk and as a surrogate to demonstrate the benefits of therapeutic interventions. B-mode ultrasound techniques to measure the intima media thickness (IMT) of the common carotid (near and far wall) and the internal carotid arteries have been fairly well standardized (Figure 7.5). Although the far wall of the common carotid is the easiest and most standardized of the measurements, most epidemiologic studies have found that a combined score of the near and far wall of the common carotid plus the internal carotid is the best predictor of CHD risk. The Cardiovascular Health Study showed that IMT at the adjustment for other risk factors was significantly associated with risk of MI and stroke. One study showed that each 0.1-mm increase in common carotid IMT is associated with a 1.91 total risk of CHD. In patients with documented CHD, the Cholesterol-Lowering Atherosclerosis Study (CLAS) showed that each 0.03-mm increase per year in carotid IMT conferred a relative risk of 2.2 for non-fatal MI or coronary death and 3.1 for any cardiovascular event.[39] Therefore, carotid IMT screening may be useful to predict increased risk in patients without documented CHD and may also be a helpful guide to intensity treatment if the IMT continues to progress. The small changes in carotid IMT (0.03-mm increase per year) that

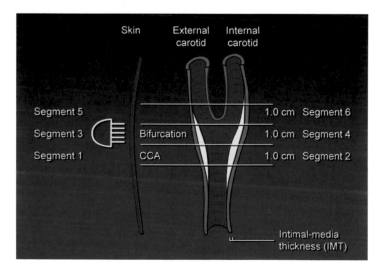

Figure 7.5   Carotid intima media thickness methodology

predict increased risk for events may be difficult to visualize unless the ultrasonography is well standardized. In the patients who continue to have progression of carotid IMT thickness, more aggressive LDL treatment or evaluation of other risk factors may be necessary. The Atorvastatin Simvastatin Atherosclerosis Project (ASAP) trial comparing simvastatin, 40 mg, to atorvastatin, 80 mg, in patients with familial hypercholesterolemia has demonstrated that in the simvastatin-treated patients, the carotid IMT continued to progress, but in the more aggressive LDL-treated group with atorvastatin, there was slight regression.[40] This study highlights the potential ability of carotid IMT measurements as a useful tool to adequately treat patients with preclinical atherosclerosis.

One of the most popular, but also perhaps the most controversial, non-invasive measures of preclinical atherosclerosis is the electron beam computed tomography (EBCT) measurement of coronary calcification.[41-42] Coronary calcification can be detected by means of traditional spiral CT scans, but these scanners use technology that is too slow to obtain clear and motionless pictures of the heart. EBCT provides image acquisition rapidly (50 to 100 milliseconds per slice) to accurately detect the coronary calcium density and volume. Coronary calcium accumulates at a relatively late stage in the atherosclerotic plaque development.

Coronary calcification is quantitated via a score calculated according to the Agatston method.[43] The area of a calcified plaque is multiplied by a coefficient estimated on the basis of the peak density of the calcified lesion. For a density of 130 to 200 Hounsfield units, the density coefficient is 1, for 201 to 300 it is 2, for 301 to 400 it is 3, and for greater than or equal to 401 the density coefficient is 4. A calcium score greater than 300 or 400 generally indicates the need for a cardiac stress test to rule out significant ischemia. Nomograms of calcium scores obtained by submitting symptomatic individuals to EBCT screening indicate the expected distribution of coronary calcification in the general population. In one study, Raggi et al published tables of calcium score percentiles derived from scoring 9728 individuals asymptomatic for coronary artery disease.[44-45] Men demonstrate a rapid increase in prevalence and extent of coronary calcification after age 40 years. In women, in contrast, calcium scores increase slowly compared to men, and a significant growth is not seen until approximately 10 years later. Furthermore, the calcium score values in women never reach the same extent as in men. The main controversy regarding the use of EBCT scanning is whether the presence of coronary calcium can be a better predictor of events than the Framingham risk score. A study was conducted in a group of 491 patients with chest pain symptoms who were submitted to sequential cardiac catheterization and EBCT imaging. After a follow-up time of 30 ± 13 months, 13 deaths and eight non-fatal MIs were recorded, and patients with a score above the median (median = 75.3) showed a risk 6-fold greater than those below the median. In logistic regression analyses that included age, gender, the number of angiographically diseased vessels, and log calcium score, the latter was the only independent predictor of an event. However, another trial evaluating younger patients demonstrated an independent effect of a high calcium score (>300) in combination with the Framingham score.

In a second study performed by the same investigators in a group of 1196 high-risk, older, and asymptomatic individuals, the predictive ability of coronary calcium scores was no greater than that of conventional risk factors.

However, the use of a suboptimal imaging protocol, which could cause the loss of significant imaging information in a group of patients already at high risk of events because of the presence of multiple risk factors, weakened the conclusions of this study.

In a study by Raggi et al the authors followed 632 asymptomatic patients screened by EBCT for an average of 3 years. At the end of the follow-up period, 19 MIs and eight deaths were recorded. Events were clustered in patients demonstrating a calcium score in the upper quartile for age and gender. Furthermore, the event rate in the upper quartile of calcium score percentile was approximately 20 times higher than in the lowest quartile, whereas the event rate in the upper quartile of risk factors was 6 times higher than in the lowest group.[46] Therefore, the hazard ratio was much larger for relative calcium score differences than for cardiovascular risk factor groups.

EBCT screening is probably best used in asymptomatic individuals at intermediate to high risk of coronary artery disease to assess the presence and extent of atherosclerotic disease and to follow up the progression of disease. Screening is best suited for particular age groups. Specifically, men should probably undergo screening between the ages of 30 and 35 years and 55 to 60 years. However, for women, screening could be useful in almost any patient older than age 40 years.

Because the Framingham risk score is a proven equation to predict CHD events and the coronary calcium score percentile for age also appears to independently predict CHD events, perhaps combining the two scores would improve the risk predictability of each score used independently. Grundy has proposed adjusting the Framingham age score based on the coronary calcium percentile for age.[47] The rationale for this adjustment is that the coronary calcium score may more effectively predict CHD events than the biologic age. As more data accumulate regarding the CHD predictive value of EBCT, it is hoped that the combination of the Framingham score with the calcium score will provide a clinically useful enhancement of risk predictability.

In addition to ABI, carotid IMT, and coronary calcium by EBCT, there are other emerging measures of preclinical disease that may provide clinical value. Perhaps the most promising is brachial artery endothelial reactivity. This non-invasive method involves the use of high-resolution ultrasound to measure changes in brachial artery diameter in response to increased flow induced by reactive hyperemia after 5 minutes of cuff occlusion of the brachial artery. In normal arteries lined by healthy endothelium, the increased flow causes dilatation of the brachial artery comparable to a sublingual nitroglycerin control. If endothelial dysfunction is present, however, the brachial artery does not dilate normally, and this impairment can be measured by ultrasound. This technique requires some skill, and the variability and interpretation have not been well standardized. Although some data have linked brachial artery reactivity to the presence of CHD, data are lacking as to whether an abnormal test predicts CHD events or an improvement in the vasodilatation correlates with a reduction in CHD rates.

As the data regarding the use of non-invasive measures of preclinical atherosclerosis continue to evolve, these tests should help determine which patients may benefit most from risk factor modification. The National Institutes of Health has launched the Multi-Ethnic Study of Atherosclerosis to help determine the most cost-effective measures or the best combination of measures to efficiently identify patients at the highest risk of clinical disease outcomes.

REFERENCES

1. Seed M, Doherty E and Stubbs P. Lipoprotein(a): a prothrombotic risk factor for coronary artery disease. J Cardiovasc Risk 1995;2: 206-21.
2. Stubbs P, Seed M, Lane D et al. Lipoprotein(a) as a risk predictor for cardiac mortality in patients with acute coronary syndromes. Eur Heart J 1998;19: 1355-64.
3. Morrisett JD. The role of lipoprotein(a) in atherosclerosis. Curr Atheroscler Rep 2000; 2: 243-50.
4. Marcovina SM, Hegele RA, Koschinsky ML. Lipoprotein(a) and coronary heart disease risk. Curr Cardiol Rep 1999;1: 105-11.
5. Austin MA, King MC, Vranizan KM et al. Atherogenic lipoprotein phenotype. A proposed genetic marker for coronary heart disease risk. Circulation 1990; 82: 495-506.
6. Angelin B. Therapy for lowering lipoprotein(a) levels. Curr Opin Lipidol 1997; 8: 337-41.
7. Brown G, Albers JJ, Fisher LD et al. Regression of coronary artery disease as a result of intensive lipid-lowering therapy in men with high levels of apolipoprotein(b). N Engl J Med 1990; 323:1289-98.
8. Herrington DM, Klein KP. Statins, hormones, and women: benefits and drawbacks for atherosclerosis and osteoporosis. Curr Atheroscler Rep 2000;3: 35-42.
9. Herrington DM, Reboussin DM, Brosnihan KB et al. Effects of estrogen replacement on the progression of coronary-artery atherosclerosis. N Engl J Med 2000; 343: 522-9.
10. Rossouw JE. Debate: the potential role of estrogen in the prevention of heart disease in women after menopause. Curr Atheroscler Rep 2000;1: 135-8.
11. Boushey CJ, Beresford SA, Omenn GS et al. A quantitative assessment of plasma homocysteine as a risk factor for vascular disease. JAMA 1995;274: 1049-57.
12. Giles WH, Crost JB, Greenlund KJ et al. Association between total homocysteine and the likelihood for a history of acute myocardial infarction by race and ethnicity: results from the Third National Health and Nutrition Examination Survey. Am Heart J 2000;139: 446-53.
13. Stehouwer CD, Weijenberg MP, van den Berg M et al. Serum homocysteine and risk of coronary heart disease and cerebrovascular disease in elderly men: a 10-year follow-up. Arterioscler Thromb Vasc Biol 1998;18: 1895-901.
14. Koenig W, Sund M, Frohlich M et al. C-reactive protein, a sensitive marker of inflammation, predicts future risk of coronary heart disease in initially healthy middle-aged men: results from the MONICA (Monitoring Trends and Determinants in Cardiovascular Disease) Augsburg Cohort Study, 1984-1992. Circulation 1999;99: 237-42.
15. Mendall MA, Strachan DP, Butland BK et al. C-reactive protein: relation to total mortality, cardiovascular mortality and cardiovascular risk factors in men. Eur Heart J 2000;21: 1584-90.
16. Ridker PM, Buring JE, Shih J et al. Prospective study of C-reactive protein and the risk of future cardiovascular events among apparently healthy women. Circulation 1998;98: 731-3.
17. Ridker PM, Glynn RJ, Hennekens CH. C-reactive protein adds to the predictive value of total and HDL cholesterol in determining risk of first myocardial infarction. Circulation 1998;97: 2007-11.
18. Ridker PM, Hennekens CH, Buring JE et al. C-reactive protein and other markers of inflammation in the prediction of cardiovascular disease in women. N Engl J Med 2000; 342: 836-43.
19. Downs JR et al Primary prevention of acute coronary events with lovastatin in men and women with average cholesterol levels: Results of the AFCAPS/TexCAPS. JAMA 1998;279: 1615 22.
20. Third Report of the National Cholesterol Education Program (NCEP) Expert Panel on Detection, Evaluation, and Treatment of High Blood Cholesterol in Adults (Adult Treatment Panel III) Final Report. Circulation 2002;106: 3143-3421.
21. Ridker PM on behalf of the JUPITER Study Group. Rosuvastatin in the primary prevention of cardiovascular disease among patients with low levels of low-density lipoprotein cholesterol and elevated high-sensitivity C-reactive protein. Rationale and design of the JUPITER trial. Circulation 2003;108: 2292-97.
22. Pearson TA, Mensah GA, Alexander RW et al. Markers of Inflammation and Cardiovascular Disease. Application to Clinical and Public Health Practice: A Statement for Healthcare

Professionals. From the Centers for Disease Control and Prevention and the American Heart Association. Circulation 2003;107: 499.

23. Ridker PM, Rifai N, Rose L et al. Comparison of C-reactive protein and low-density lipoprotein cholesterol levels in the prediction of first cardiovascular events. N Engl J Med 2002;347:1557–65.

24. Budde T, Fechtrup C, Bosenberg E et al. Plasma Lp(a) levels correlate with number, severity, and length-extension of coronary lesions in male patients undergoing coronary arteriography for clinically suspected coronary atherosclerosis. Arterioscler Thromb 1994;14: 1730–6.

25. HYPERLINK "http://www.lipidsonline.org/redirect.cfm?link=http%3A%2F%2Fwww%2Encbi%2Enlm%2Enih%2Egov%2Fentrez%2Fquery%2Efcgi%3Fcmd%3DRetrieve%26db%3DPubMed%26list%5Fuids%3D7566020%26dopt%3DAbstract" \t "ref" Shepherd J, Cobbe SM, Ford I, et al. Prevention of coronary heart disease with pravastatin in men with hypercholesterolemia. N Engl J Med 1995;333: 1301-7.

26. Buring JE, Hennekens CH for the Women's Health Study Research Group. The Women's Health Study: rationale and background. J Myo Isch 1992;4: 30-40.

27. Chambless LE, Heiss G, Folsom AR et al. Association of coronary heart disease incidence with carotid arterial wall thickness and major risk factors: the Atherosclerosis Risk in Communities (ARIC) Study. Am J Epidemiol 1997;146: 483–94.

28. Tunstall-Pedoe H for the WHO MONICA Project. The World Health Organization MONICA Project (Monitoring Trends and Determinants in Cardiovascular Disease): A major international collaboration. J Clin Epidemiol 1988;41: 105-14.

29. TIMI Study Group The thrombolysis in myocardial infarction (TIMI) trial: Phase I findings. New Engl J Med 1985;312: 932-6.

30. Shepherd J, Blauw GJ, Murphy MB, et al, on behalf of the PROSPER study group. Pravastatin in elderly individuals at risk of vascular disease (PROSPER): a randomized controlled trial. Lancet 2002;360: 1623-30.

31. Psaty BM, Furberg CD, Kuller LH et al Traditional risk factors and subclinical disease measures as predictors of first myocardial infarction in older adults: the Cardiovascular Health Study. Arch Intern Med 1999;159: 1339-47.

32. Barrett-Connor E. Hypercholesterolemia predicts early death from coronary heart disease in elderly men but not women. The Rancho Bernardo Study. Ann Epidemiol 1992;2: 77-83.

33. Lahmann PH et al. A Prospective Study of Adiposity and All-Cause Mortality: The Malmö Diet and Cancer Study. Obesity Research 2002;10: 361-69.

34. Otvos JD, Jeyarajah EJ, Cromwell WC. Measurement issues related to lipoprotein heterogeneity. Am J Cardiol 2002;90: 22i-29i.

35. Despres JP, Lamarche B, Mauriege P et al. Hyperinsulinemia as an independent risk factor for ischemic heart disease. N Eng J Med 1996;334: 952-7.

36. Leng GC, Fowkes FG, Lee AJ et al. Use of ankle brachial pressure index to predict cardiovascular events and death: a cohort study. BMJ 1996;313: 1440-4.

37. McKenna M, Wolfson S, Kuller L. The ratio of ankle and arm arterial pressure as an independent predictor of mortality. Atherosclerosis 1991;87: 119–28.

38. Mann JF, Gerstein HC, Pogue J et al. Renal insufficiency as a predictor of cardiovascular outcomes and the impact of ramipril: the HOPE Randomized Trial. Ann Int Med 2001; 134: 629-36.

39. Blankenhorn DH, Alaupovic P, Wickham E et al. Prediction of angiographic change in native human coronary arteries and aortocoronary bypass grafts. Lipid and nonlipid factors. Circulation 1990;81: 470-76.

40. Smilde TJ, Wissen S, Wollersheim H et al. Effect of aggressive versus conventional lipid lowering on atherosclerosis progression in familial hypercholesterolaemia (ASAP): a prospective, randomized, double-blind trial. Lancet 2001;357: 577–81.

41. O'Rourke RA, Brundage BH, Froelicher VF et al. American College of Cardiology/American Heart Association Expert Consensus document on electron-beam computed tomography for the diagnosis and prognosis of coronary artery disease. Circulation 2000;102: 126–40.

42. Raggi P. Electron beam tomography as an endpoint for clinical trials of anti-atherosclerotic therapy. Curr Atheroscler Rep 2000;2: 284–9.
43. Agatston AS et al. Quantification of coronary artery calcium using ultrafast computerized tomography. J Am Coll Cardiol 1990;15: 827-32.
44. Raggi P, Shaw LJ, Berman DS et al. Gender-based differences in the prognostic value of coronary calcification. J Women's Health 2004;13: 273-83.
45. Raggi P. Prognostic implications of absolute and relative calcium scores. Herz 2001; 26: 252-9.
46. Raggi P, Callister TQ, Cooil B et al. Identification of patients at increased risk of first unheralded acute myocardial infarction by electron-beam computed tomography. Circulation 2000;101: 850–5.
47. Grundy SM, Bazzarre T, Cleeman J et al. Prevention Conference V: Beyond secondary prevention: identifying the high-risk patient for primary prevention: medical office assessment: Writing Group I. Circulation 2000;101: E3–11.

8

Clinical signs of atherosclerosis

Barbara C Biedermann

Introduction • Cardiovascular risk scores: strengths and limitations
• The family history: a simple 'genetic' test • Bedside procedures
to assess cardiovascular disease • Conclusion

INTRODUCTION

Atherosclerosis is a common and global disease.[1] Its prevalence increases with age. In the primary care setting, 12–14% of patients suffer from symptomatic atherosclerosis[2,3] compared to 45% in hospitalized patients.[4] Among the latter patient population, up to 80% of individuals in the ninth decade have a history of previous cardiovascular events due to atherosclerosis. The disease affects the large arteries, including the aortic tree and its major branches (Figure 8.1). Common cardiovascular events occur in different vascular beds and are a sign of coronary heart disease, cerebrovascular disease, peripheral arterial disease, aortic or renovascular disease. Atherosclerosis is a panarterial disease and specific morphologic signs of the disease occur in all vascular beds examined.[1] Atherosclerotic lesions, the so called 'plaques', form in the arterial wall.[5]

Atherosclerosis remains clinically silent until organ ischemia causes symptoms (Figure 8.2). The term 'vulnerable patient'[6,7] has been coined to emphasize this transition and to concentrate preventive efforts on the presymptomatic stage of the disease. It is very important to distinguish the symptomatic, malign from the asymptomatic, benign course of the disease. Early stages of the disease such as fatty streaks occur at a young age.[8] Acute arterial obstruction is usually caused by plaque rupture or erosion followed by arterial thrombosis,[9] and precipitates cardiovascular events such as myocardial infarction, stroke, or painful leg ischemia. In the general population, the prevalence of coronary heart disease is 7.8% and of cerebrovascular or peripheral arterial occlusive disease 3.1 or 3.8%, respectively.[3] Chronic arterial obstruction leads to more insidious symptoms such as angina pectoris, heart failure, dementia, renal failure, renal hypertension, or claudication in the lower extremities. At the end of life, 85% of individuals have developed significant atherosclerotic plaques but only half of them have ever suffered from cardiovascular events (Figure 8.2). Only 10–15% of individuals neither develop atherosclerotic plaques nor cardiovascular events during their lifetime.[4]

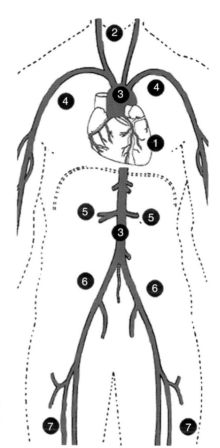

Figure 8.1 The human arterial tree. 1) coronary arteries. 2) carotid arteries. 3) aorta. 4) subclavian arteries. 5) renal arteries. 6) iliac arteries. 7) femoral arteries.

In order to effectively prevent symptomatic disease, it is important to identify vulnerable individuals before events occur and before the more insidious, chronic course of atherosclerosis leads to progressive disability. This would open a *window of opportunity* to treat the patient in a presymptomatic state. The individual probability to develop atherosclerosis is determined by environmental injury and genetic predisposition. Several clinical scores have been developed to assess the individual risk, i.e. the probability for cardiovascular events to occur over a certain period of time.[10–12] Some of the traditional cardiovascular risk factors like smoking, diabetes mellitus, arterial hypertension, or hypercholesterolemia are completely or partially influenced by lifestyle or environment. Several Scandinavian twin studies have shown significant differences in the concordance rate of cardiovascular events in monozygotic and dizygotic twins,[13] proving that atherosclerosis has a genetic background. The genetic impact on the course of the disease as determined by twin studies is detectable in younger subjects and disappears at more advanced age, i.e. >75 years.[14] Single gene polymorphisms (SNPs) that are associated with arteriosclerosis have generally a weak penetrance, i.e. the percentage of SNP carriers that develop disease is low.[15] A positive

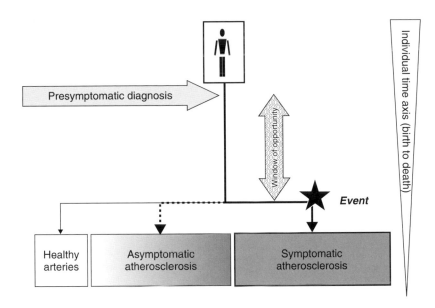

Figure 8.2   The lifetime incidence of atherosclerotic lesion formation and cardiovascular events.

family history for cardiovascular events provides more comprehensive evidence for the genetic predisposition of an individual to develop atherosclerosis.

Finally, not all individuals with risk factors or genetic susceptibility develop disease. The lifelong treatment of patients who do not require or do not profit from a therapy should be avoided to maintain quality of life and to reduce health economic burden. The reliable assessment of clinical disease activity and plaque burden is of decisive importance to reach this goal. Ideally it should be based on a set of available, simple, accurate, affordable, and non invasive clinical procedures. The medical physical examination fulfills these criteria very well, but is often neglected in modern medicine. Pedal pulse palpation, auscultation of the arterial tree for vascular bruits, and the ankle brachial index (ABI) are bedside procedures to identify individuals with clinically significant atherosclerosis. This chapter will discuss the value of clinical risk scores, family history and bedside procedures as non-invasive surrogate markers of atherosclerosis (Figure 8.3).

CARDIOVASCULAR RISK SCORES: STRENGTHS AND LIMITATIONS

This section does not aim to give a complete and balanced overview of the vast published literature about cardiovascular risk factor assessment tools, but rather wishes to discuss the value and limitation of this approach to improve an individual patient's care. Risk scores have been developed to accurately predict individual risk and to implement best proven therapy in patients threatened by cardiovascular events.[10, 11] They are particularly useful in the setting of primary prevention. Published evidence that validates these risk scores enters the official

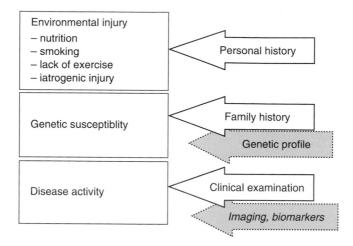

Figure 8.3   Basic clinical methods to diagnose (presymptomatic) atherosclerosis.

guidelines of the political health authorities that are updated on a regular basis.[16-19] Gender, age, smoking habits, diabetes, blood pressure, total cholesterol, low-density lipoprotein (LDL) and high-density lipoprotein (HDL) cholesterol usually enter these algorithms for disease prediction.[20]

As an example, the individual risk estimate according to the New Zealand guidelines on management of dyslipidemia[12] and raised blood pressure[18] is discussed here. Based on an individual patient's values, his risk level is assessed to be very high (>20% probability to develop cardiovascular events in 5 years), high (15–20%), moderate (10–15%), or low (>10%). The benefit of a therapeutic intervention (i.e. lowering total cholesterol by 20%, systolic blood pressure by 10–15 mmHg, or diastolic blood pressure by 5–10 mmHg) to prevent cardiovascular events over the next 5 years is quantified by the number needed to treat (NNT). The NNT is less than 13 patients in the 'very high' and higher than 40 in the 'low' risk group. A value of 13 for the NNT is good for a primary preventive intervention, but it still means that 12 of 13 individuals receive treatment without personal benefit.

Although helpful for the management of high-risk individuals in a primary prevention setting, there are some limitations to the general applicability of these cardiovascular risk scores. First, risk assessment within a given population strongly varies with the guideline that is used.[20-23] A Canadian study[23] recently compared Canadian, US, EU, British, Australian, and New Zealand guidelines for the efficiency (measured by the NNT) and effectiveness (i.e. the potential number of deaths from coronary heart disease prevented if all community members were screened by the respective guideline) of statin treatment in primary prevention. The NNT was 108 or 198, respectively, when the New Zealand guidelines or the US guidelines were applied. Furthermore, the percentage of the population that required statin treatment to prevent a similar number of deaths varied between 12.9 and 24.5% when different guidelines were applied. Remarkably, in this study on Canadian individuals, the Canadian guidelines provided neither the most effective nor the most efficient rules to identify the patients at risk. The second limitation of risk scores results from the fact that some of the variables that are part of the risk prediction algorithms, e.g. blood pressure or cholesterol, change with treatment. Therefore, most of the risk prediction scores apply to the untreated, free-living subjects only.[11] Third, guidelines are usually focused on one organ system that is affected by cardiovascular events, e.g. the heart or the brain. Since myocardial infarction and stroke are common and well defined entities, most of the clinical trials are actually validated for the prevention of these two cardiovascular events, including cardiovascular death. As outlined in the introduction, although atherosclerosis is essentially a panarterial disease,[4] plaque burden in the coronary, the carotid, the renal, and peripheral arteries varies significantly,[24] and the pathogenic mechanism of ischemic cardiovascular events may be distinct in the different organs.[9, 25] Therefore, it may not be justified to use treatment recommendations that were established to prevent coronary heart disease for the management of cerebrovascular or peripheral arterial occlusive disease.

THE FAMILY HISTORY: A SIMPLE 'GENETIC' TEST

Twin studies have shown that cardiovascular events are more common in monozygotic (39% in men, 44% in women) than in dizygotic twins (29% in men, 14% in women).[26] These concordance rates suggest that atherosclerosis has a strong genetic background. Except for a few monogenetic disorders[27] with high penetrance for symptomatic atherosclerosis (e.g. familial hypercholesterolemia due to LDL receptor mutations), most genetic polymorphisms that were reported to be associated with symptomatic atherosclerosis have low penetrance, reflected by low OR.[28–33] In a Japanese study, a selection of 71 candidate genes was screened for 112 known SNPs in 909 subjects, half of them with myocardial infarction. In a larger confirmational study, focusing on the most promising SNPs associated with symptomatic atherosclerosis, connexin 37 (C1019T) and p22^{phox} (C242T) had odds ratios of 1.4 and 0.7, respectively, for myocardial infarction in men ($n = 2858$). In women ($n = 1294$), different SNPs were most closely associated with myocardial infarction: PAI type 1 (4G-668/5G) and stromelysin-1 (5A-1171/6A) had an OR of 1.6 and 4.7, respectively, for symptomatic atherosclerosis. The disappointingly low diagnostic and predictive value of genetic tests that identify common polymorphisms is paralleled or exceeded by a positive family history.[34,35] The OR for cardiovascular disease to occur within 8 years is 2.33 for subjects with siblings affected by the disease and 3.2 (for men) and 2.9 (for women), for subjects with one or two parents suffering from premature atherosclerosis. When both parents are affected, the OR for men is 5.2 (corresponding to a probability of 83% to suffer an event). Similar data are obtained for non-premature atherosclerosis.[35] In a prospective analysis investigating aortic elastance as a non-invasive surrogate marker of atherosclerosis, positive family history had an OR of 2.59 for cardiovascular events as the novel test under investigation.[36] Therefore, positive family history has an equivalent or even superior diagnostic and predictive value to any single genetic polymorphism tested so far.

BEDSIDE PROCEDURES TO ASSESS CARDIOVASCULAR DISEASE

A complete general physical examination should always be performed in a patient with suspected cardiovascular disease. Pedal pulse palpation, auscultation for vascular bruits and the ABI have been selected here as validated clinical tests for the diagnosis of atherosclerosis.

Abnormal pedal pulses are quite sensitive and specific for the diagnosis of clinically-significant atherosclerosis of the lower extremity (for review see reference 37). Sensitivity varies between 63 and 95% and specificity between 99 and 73%, respectively, depending on the clinical setting.[38–40]

A vascular murmur is the most immediate physical sign of an arterial stenosis. The diagnostic value of careful auscultation for vascular bruits is well established for the carotid, the abdominal, and the peripheral arteries (Table 8.1). The physician's clinical experience clearly improves diagnostic accuracy of these simple clinical procedures.[41] The sensitivity of detectable systolic vascular murmurs for the diagnosis of atherosclerosis is significantly high in the carotid and the renal arteries, but it is disappointingly low in the femoral artery as a consequence of low blood flow at rest. Therefore, the sensitivity of the test can be improved with exercise, e.g. repetitive toe stands. For the carotid artery, using angiography as the gold standard method, the sensitivity and specificity of systolic carotid bruits are different in asymptomatic (sensitivity 90%, specificity 86%[42]) compared to symptomatic (sensitivity 62%, specificity 61%[43]) patients. This is unexpected since high pretest probability usually improves the diagnostic accuracy of a test.

The ABI is the third clinical test suitable for the direct assessment of arterial health. It is less observer-dependent than auscultation and palpation and is still available as a simple, inexpensive bedside procedure with high acceptance in primary care physicians.[3] Based on the principle that atherosclerotic plaques in the iliac, femoral or popliteal arteries limit flow to the lower leg arteries, the blood pressure difference between the arm and the ankle is detected.[44] The procedure is not uniformly described in the published literature. Generally, blood pressure is measured in both upper extremities and the higher of the two blood pressures is taken to divide the ankle blood pressure. The systolic ankle

Table 8.1 Sensitivity and specificity of systolic vascular bruits for the diagnosis of atherosclerotic arterial stenosis

Vascular bed	Sensitivity %	Specificity %	Reference
Carotid artery			
asymptomatic patients	90	86	42
	58	88	47
symptomatic patients	62	61	43
	71	79	48
Renal artery	39	99	49
	63	90	50
Femoral artery	20	96	51
	29	95	40

blood pressure is detected by measuring flow with hand-held Doppler in the dorsal pedal and posterior tibial artery when the blood pressure cuff is inflated around the ankle. The blood pressure at which the Doppler signal disappears in the two arteries is registered and the higher of the two values enters the formula. Generally, a value ≤ 0.9 is considered abnormal and indicates relevant peripheral arterial disease.[44] For the diagnosis of peripheral arterial occlusive disease, an abnormal ABI has been reported to have a specificity of 100% and a sensitivity of 97%.[45] For the accurate non-invasive diagnosis of peripheral arterial disease, ABI is superior to treadmill exercise or postocclusive reactive hyperemia.[45] However, for the diagnosis of atherosclerosis as a panarterial disease, sensitivity is substantially lower. In a systematic review including four population-based clinical studies that correlated abnormal ABI with cardiovascular outcome, i.e. death by myocardial infarction or stroke, specificity was 87.9% and sensitivity 41%.[46]

CONCLUSION

The assessment of the cardiovascular risk factors, the determination of the individual cardiovascular risk, and a positive familiy history for symptomatic atherosclerosis are not diagnostic procedures in the strict sense. The probability to develop cardiovascular events in the near future is considered to be 'very high' when it exceeds 20%. This means that still 80% of the individuals with this risk will remain free of an event. Since symptomatic atherosclerosis is increasingly common with age, the probability of asymptomatic individuals above 70 to suffer cardiovascular events is always estimated to be 'very high'. Risk scores lose their stratifying strength in this age group. In contrast, pedal pulse palpation, auscultation of arterial sites, and ABI are diagnostic procedures for atherosclerotic disease, and the sensitivity and specificity for these tests have been determined in several independent clinical trials. The specificity for these three bedside tests is reasonably good, but sensitivity to exclude atherosclerosis as a panarterial disease is insufficient. In order to focus treatment of atherosclerosis on the patients who need it and who will respond to therapy, diagnostic procedures with higher sensitivity are required to identify presymptomatic disease.

REFERENCES

1. Yusuf S, Hawken S, Ounpuu S et al. Obesity and the risk of myocardial infarction in 27,000 participants from 52 countries: a case-control study. Lancet 2005; 366(9497): 1640–9.
2. McDermott MM, Kerwin DR, Liu K et al. Prevalence and significance of unrecognized lower extremity peripheral arterial disease in general medicine practice. J Gen Intern Med 2001; 16(6): 384–90.
3. Hayoz D, Bounameaux H, Canova CR. Swiss Athcrothrombosis Survey: a field report on the occurrence of symptomatic and asymptomatic peripheral arterial disease. J Intern Med 2005; 258(3): 238–43.
4. Fleiner M, Kummer M, Mirlacher M et al. Arterial neovascularization and inflammation in vulnerable patients: early and late signs of symptomatic atherosclerosis. Circulation 2004; 110(18): 2843–50.
5. Stary HC, Chandler AB, Dinsmore RE et al. A definition of advanced types of atherosclerotic lesions and a histological classification of atherosclerosis. A report from the Committee on Vascular Lesions of the Council on Arteriosclerosis, American Heart Association. Circulation 1995; 92(5): 1355–74.

6. Naghavi M, Libby P, Falk E et al. From vulnerable plaque to vulnerable patient: a call for new definitions and risk assessment strategies: Part I. Circulation 2003; 108(14): 1664–72.
7. Naghavi M, Libby P, Falk E et al. From vulnerable plaque to vulnerable patient: a call for new definitions and risk assessment strategies: Part II. Circulation 2003; 108(15): 1772–8.
8. Strong JP, Malcom GT, McMahan CA et al. Prevalence and extent of atherosclerosis in adolescents and young adults: implications for prevention from the Pathobiological Determinants of Atherosclerosis in Youth Study. JAMA 1999; 281(8): 727–35.
9. Virmani R, Kolodgie FD, Burke AP et al. Lessons from sudden coronary death: a comprehensive morphological classification scheme for atherosclerotic lesions. Arterioscler Thromb Vasc Biol 2000; 20(5): 1262–75.
10. Assmann G, Cullen P, Schulte H. Simple scoring scheme for calculating the risk of acute coronary events based on the 10-year follow-up of the prospective cardiovascular Munster (PROCAM) study. Circulation 2002; 105(3): 310–15.
11. Wilson PW, D'Agostino RB, Levy D et al. Prediction of coronary heart disease using risk factor categories. Circulation 1998; 97(18): 1837–47.
12. 1996 National Heart Foundation clinical guidelines for the assessment and management of dyslipidaemia. Dyslipidaemia Advisory Group on behalf of the scientific committee of the National Heart Foundation of New Zealand. NZ Med J 1996; 109(1024): 224–31.
13. Scheuner MT. Genetic predisposition to coronary artery disease. Curr Opin Cardiol 2001; 16(4): 251–60.
14. Marenberg ME, Risch N, Berkman LF et al. Genetic susceptibility to death from coronary heart disease in a study of twins. N Engl J Med 1994; 330(15): 1041–6.
15. Yamada Y, Izawa H, Ichihara S, et al. Prediction of the risk of myocardial infarction from polymorphisms in candidate genes. N Engl J Med 2002; 347(24): 1916–23.
16. Smith SC, Jr., Allen J, Blair SN et al. AHA/ACC guidelines for secondary prevention for patients with coronary and other atherosclerotic vascular disease: 2006 update: endorsed by the National Heart, Lung, and Blood Institute. Circulation 2006; 113(19): 2363–72.
17. De Backer G, Ambrosioni E, Borch-Johnsen K et al. European guidelines on cardiovascular disease prevention in clinical practice. Third Joint Task Force of European and Other Societies on Cardiovascular Disease Prevention in Clinical Practice. Eur Heart J 2003; 24(17): 1601–10.
18. New Zealand Guidelines Group, 2003. http://www.nzgg.org.nz/guidelines/0035/CVD_Risk_Full.pdf.
19. British Heart Foundation, 2004. http://www.bhf.org.uk/professionals/uploaded/aug_2004%20v2.pdf.
20. Broedl UC, Geiss HC, Parhofer KG. Comparison of current guidelines for primary prevention of coronary heart disease: risk assessment and lipid-lowering therapy. J Gen Intern Med 2003; 18(3): 190–5.
21. Empana JP, Ducimetiere P, Arveiler D et al. Are the Framingham and PROCAM coronary heart disease risk functions applicable to different European populations? The PRIME Study. Eur Heart J 2003; 24(21): 1903–11.
22. Lengele JP, Vinck WJ, De Plaen JF et al. Cardiovascular risk assessment in hypertensive patients: major discrepancy according to ESH and SCORE strategies. J Hypertens 2007; 25(4): 757–62.
23. Manuel DG, Kwong K, Tanuseputro P et al. Effectiveness and efficiency of different guidelines on statin treatment for preventing deaths from coronary heart disease: modelling study. BMJ 2006; 332(7555): 1419.
24. Wyler von Ballmoos M, Dubler D, Mirlacher M et al. Increased apolipoprotein deposits in early atherosclerotic lesions distinguish symptomatic from asymptomatic patients. Arterioscler Thromb Vasc Biol 2006; 26(2): 359–64.
25. Redgrave JN, Lovett JK, Gallagher PJ et al. Histological assessment of 526 symptomatic carotid plaques in relation to the nature and timing of ischemic symptoms: the Oxford plaque study. Circulation 2006; 113(19): 2320–8.
26. Allen G, Harvald B, Shields J. Measures of twin concordance. Acta Genet Stat Med 1967; 17(6): 475–81.

27. Goldstein JL, Brown MS. Molecular medicine. The cholesterol quartet. Science 2001; 292(5520): 1310–12.
28. Clee SM, Zwinderman AH, Engert JC et al. Common genetic variation in ABCA1 is associated with altered lipoprotein levels and a modified risk for coronary artery disease. Circulation 2001; 103(9): 1198–205.
29. Wittrup HH, Tybjaerg-Hansen A, Steffensen R et al. Mutations in the lipoprotein lipase gene associated with ischemic heart disease in men. The Copenhagen city heart study. Arterioscler Thromb Vasc Biol 1999; 19(6): 1535–40.
30. Inoue N, Kawashima S, Kanazawa K et al. Polymorphism of the NADH/NADPH oxidase p22 phox gene in patients with coronary artery disease. Circulation 1998; 97(2): 135–7.
31. Humphries SE, Martin S, Cooper J et al. Interaction between smoking and the stromelysin-1 (MMP3) gene 5A/6A promoter polymorphism and risk of coronary heart disease in healthy men. Ann Hum Genet 2002; 66(Pt 5–6): 343–52.
32. Frosst P, Blom HJ, Milos R et al. A candidate genetic risk factor for vascular disease: a common mutation in methylenetetrahydrofolate reductase. Nat Genet 1995; 10(1): 111–13.
33. Ye SQ, Usher D, Virgil D et al. A PstI polymorphism detects the mutation of serine128 to arginine in CD 62E gene – a risk factor for coronary artery disease. J Biomed Sci 1999; 6(1): 18–21.
34. Murabito JM, Pencina MJ, Nam BH et al. Sibling cardiovascular disease as a risk factor for cardiovascular disease in middle-aged adults. JAMA 2005; 294(24): 3117–23.
35. Lloyd-Jones DM, Nam BH, D'Agostino RB, Sr., Levy D, Murabito JM, Wang TJ, et al. Parental cardiovascular disease as a risk factor for cardiovascular disease in middle-aged adults: a prospective study of parents and offspring. JAMA 2004; 291(18): 2204–11.
36. Hunziker PR, Imsand C, Keller D et al. Bedside quantification of atherosclerosis severity for cardiovascular risk stratification: a prospective cohort study. J Am Coll Cardiol 2002; 39(4): 702–9.
37. McGee SR, Boyko EJ. Physical examination and chronic lower-extremity ischemia: a critical review. Arch Intern Med 1998; 158(12): 1357–64.
38. Christensen JH, Freundlich M, Jacobsen BA et al. Clinical relevance of pedal pulse palpation in patients suspected of peripheral arterial insufficiency. J Intern Med 1989; 226(2): 95–9.
39. Boyko EJ, Ahroni JH, Davignon D et al. Diagnostic utility of the history and physical examination for peripheral vascular disease among patients with diabetes mellitus. J Clin Epidemiol 1997; 50(6): 659–68.
40. Stoffers HE, Kester AD, Kaiser V et al. Diagnostic value of signs and symptoms associated with peripheral arterial occlusive disease seen in general practice: a multivariable approach. Med Decis Making 1997; 17(1): 61–70.
41. Baker WH, String ST, Hayes AC et al. Diagnosis of peripheral occlusive disease: comparison of clinical evaluation and noninvasive laboratory. Arch Surg 1978; 113(11): 1308–10.
42. David TE, Humphries AW, Young JR et al. A correlation of neck bruits and arteriosclerotic carotid arteries. Arch Surg 1973; 107(5): 729–31.
43. Beneficial effect of carotid endarterectomy in symptomatic patients with high-grade carotid stenosis. North American Symptomatic Carotid Endarterectomy Trial Collaborators. N Engl J Med 1991; 325(7): 445–53.
44. Redberg RF, Vogel RA, Criqui MH et al. 34th Bethesda Conference: Task force #3 – What is the spectrum of current and emerging techniques for the noninvasive measurement of atherosclerosis? J Am Coll Cardiol 2003; 41(11): 1886–98.
45. Ouriel K, McDonnell AE, Metz CE et al. Critical evaluation of stress testing in the diagnosis of peripheral vascular disease. Surgery 1982; 91(6): 686–93.
46. Doobay AV, Anand SS. Sensitivity and specificity of the ankle-brachial index to predict future cardiovascular outcomes: a systematic review. Arterioscler Thromb Vasc Biol 2005; 25(7): 1463–9.
47. Gentile AT, Taylor LM, Jr., Moneta GL et al. Prevalence of asymptomatic carotid stenosis in patients undergoing infrainguinal bypass surgery. Arch Surg 1995; 130(8): 900–4.
48. Hankey GJ, Warlow CP. Symptomatic carotid ischaemic events: safest and most cost effective way of selecting patients for angiography, before carotid endarterectomy. BMJ 1990; 300(6738): 1485–91.

49. Grim CE, Luft FC, Weinberger MH et al. Sensitivity and specificity of screening tests for renal vascular hypertension. Ann Intern Med 1979; 91(4): 617–22.
50. Fenton SS, Lyttle JA, Pantridge JF. Diagnosis and results of surgery in renovascular hypertension. Lancet 1966; 2(7455): 117–21.
51. Criqui MH, Fronek A, Klauber MR et al. The sensitivity, specificity, and predictive value of traditional clinical evaluation of peripheral arterial disease: results from noninvasive testing in a defined population. Circulation 1985; 71(3): 516–22.

Index